The Multisensory Handbook

Do you support a child or adult with sensory perceptual issues or cognitive impairment?

For people with challenging sensory and cognitive conditions, everyday life can be so unpredictable and chaotic that, over time, lack of engagement can often lead to a state of learned helplessness. In this insightful text, Paul Pagliano shows how 'learned helplessness' can be transformed into learned optimism through multisensory stimulation, and explains how a programme of support can be designed and modulated to match a person's needs, interests and abilities. Using practical, easy-to-use multisensory assessment tools and intervention strategies, this book will help the individual to

*   foster a feeling of ease with the environment;
*   experience pleasure and happiness in their surroundings;
*   kindle their desire to explore;
*   improve their learning, social wellbeing and quality of life.

The author offers an abundance of exciting multisensory stimulation ideas that can be applied to communication, play, leisure and recreation, therapy and education. Practical resources also show how to monitor and review applications to ensure they are being used in the most effective and enjoyable ways possible.

Informed by an astute, up-to-date, comprehensive overview of research and theory, *The Multisensory Handbook* will appeal to primary professionals from a wide range of disciplines including education, health and social care.

Paul Pagliano is Associate Professor in Education at James Cook University, Australia. He has an international reputation as a public speaker, and is on the editorial boards of seven academic journals.

The Multisensory Handbook

A guide for children and adults
with sensory learning disabilities

Paul Pagliano

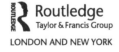
Routledge
Taylor & Francis Group

LONDON AND NEW YORK

First published 2012
by Routledge
2 Park Square, Milton Park, Abingdon, Oxon OX14 4RN

Simultaneously published in the USA and Canada
by Routledge
711 Third Avenue, New York, NY 10017

Routledge is an imprint of the Taylor & Francis Group, an informa business

© 2012 Paul Pagliano

British Library Cataloguing in Publication Data
A catalogue record for this book is available from the British Library

Library of Congress Cataloging-in-Publication Data
Pagliano, Paul J.
  The multisensory handbook : a guide for children and adults with sensory
learning disabilities / Paul Pagliano.
      p. cm.
    Includes bibliographical references and index.
  Sensory stimulation. 2. Perceptual-motor learning. 3. Perception–
Physiological aspects. 4. People with disabilities–Rehabilitation. I. Title.
  QP442.P34 2012
  616.8'4–dc23   2011049164

ISBN: 978-0-415-59754-8 (pbk)
ISBN: 978-0-203-11738-5 (ebk)

Typeset in Bembo by
Swales & Willis Ltd, Exeter, Devon

For Fiona, Zachary, Christopher and Matthew

Contents

Illustrations

Figures

Tables

Acknowledgements

The case examples in this book are fictional creations loosely based on experiences I have had in my professional career.

I would like to thank the students and staff of Kilparrin Teaching and Assessment School and Services for inviting me to be part of the learning; Dr Marja Sirkkola; Ad Verheul and Yan Hulsegge; Dr Sandra Fornes and Bud Kirschner of the Christopher Douglas Hidden Angel Foundation; Flo Longhorm, Richard and Lois Hirstwood of Florich Productions and Hirstwood Training; Dr Krista Mertens; Mauritz Eijgendaal; Dr Sue Kuhl; Elaine Gilmour; Linda Messbauer; Susanne Little; Päivi Veikkola; Michele Shapiro; my employer James Cook University; and a special thanks to my wife Dr Fiona McWhinnie 'for seeing the best in me'.

Part I

Multisensory stimulation

Chapter 1

The senses and the brain

Introduction

This book investigates multisensory stimulation particularly in the context of children and adults with sensory and learning disabilities. We begin our journey by introducing the basic terms and ideas that will be required and then follow with an overview of the importance of the senses in human development, learning, functioning and wellbeing.

Our senses connect our brains to the concrete world (including our own bodies) and they are essential for our survival. There is still much debate as to exactly how many different senses we have, whether the number is five, sixteen or even higher, and their relative importance to each other. Needless to say, we are multisensory beings and we live in a multisensory world. We have a multitude of different ways to obtain information about the world and ourselves and when this information is efficiently processed, it provides us with a tremendously rich and sophisticated understanding of the world. It is this understanding that not only enables us to determine who we are and how we live but also, because it seems to happen so automatically, affords us the luxury of taking the whole process for granted.

The situation changes dramatically if we are in an environmental circumstance or we have some physical condition that precludes us from being able to engage with these sensory stimuli. Prolonged severe sensory deprivation has pervasive negative effects on every aspect of human functioning, development and wellbeing, including in extreme cases atrophy of the brain and even death. Sensory deprivation may occur because of environmental conditions, inadequate sensory processing, or a combination of both. It may occur at any age. Whatever the cause, however, the result is the same – sensory deprivation drastically reduces opportunities for self-determination and wellbeing.

Chapter 1 introduces the key terms and makes a start on developing a rationale beginning with the first principle, which is that we naturally function best at a multisensory level so whenever possible we need to provide multisensory stimulation. This book is an exploration of multisensory stimulation and how it can be employed to help people with sense disabilities to use their senses in the most gratifying and effective ways they can.

Basic terms

These are some of the basic terms used throughout the book:

- A sense is any faculty that accesses stimuli from inside or outside the body.
- Sense stimulation is anything that triggers activity in a sense nerve receptor. Anything seen are visual stimuli, anything heard are auditory stimuli, and so on for each of the senses.
- Perception is the process of becoming aware of, recognising and interpreting the stimuli.
- Sensory processing is an umbrella term that refers to the interface where a sense ends and where perception begins, to describe the two working in combination.
- Multisensory stimulation is stimulation that simultaneously appeals to more than one set of sense nerve receptors.

Nervous system

Our nervous system has much to do in order for us to become aware of, receive, organise and interpret sensory information and then to act on it. There is a continuous flow of information from the senses, through the nervous system to the brain, and back to the body parts. The brain sorts through the sensory information it receives to gain an understanding of what is happening inside the body, what is going on outside the body, assesses how these two sets of information may be interrelated and then determines what might be the best course of action. The brain makes decisions based on the totality of this information. Some of the processing is at a conscious or voluntary level and some of it is at a subconscious or involuntary level. For example we might put our finger on something that is dangerously hot. This sense information travels from the finger to the brain and then it travels back to the finger again with an urgent instruction to move it to safety. Simultaneously other information is sent to vital body organs such as the heart to prepare them for a state of full alert.

The nervous system consists of three subsystems: the central, the peripheral and the autonomic nervous system:

1   The central nervous system (CNS) comprises the brain, spinal cord and retina. The retina is an extension of the optic nerve and therefore contiguous with the brain. It is the only sense organ that is regarded as a part of the brain.
2   The peripheral nervous system (PNS) provides the communication channels between the CNS and the rest of the body. It is made up of the sensory division, and the motor division. The sensory division is called the afferent division because it takes information to the brain, nerve fibres conduct electrical impulses to the CNS, while the motor division is called the

efferent division because it takes information away from the brain, nerve fibres conduct impulses from the CNS to the muscles.

3   The autonomic nervous system (ANS) regulates the internal environment of the person. It conducts impulses from the CNS to the internal organs and glands. The system is involuntary. The ANS has two divisions, sympathetic and parasympathetic. The sympathetic division mobilises systems during activity, for example, fight or flight, with two arousal-neurotransmitters, epinephrine and norepinephrine. The parasympathetic division is involved in stimulation of systems active during periods of rest, for example, digestion, via the neurotransmitter acetylcholine.

A simple sensory stimulus, if powerful enough, triggers a nerve receptor, which can in turn set in motion a cascade of neural electrical impulses. A complex stimulus triggers a variety of nerve receptors, which can in turn trigger an even bigger cascade of neural electrical impulses. As the information travels through the nervous system it passes through relays called synapses. Here the information can be facilitated and/or inhibited, which ultimately influences how the stimulus is cognitively perceived. The process is dynamic.

Neuroplasticity

Through the neural pathways, a sensory stimulus causes changes in the brain. This idea is called neuroplasticity. Neuroplasticity is an incredibly complex process but results in the brain changing itself depending on the amount and type of stimulation it receives. Neuroplasticity challenges the idea that brain functions are fixed in certain locations. If one part of the brain is not used then it shrinks or another part of the brain takes over. The idea of neuroplasticity is a dynamic process that starts with Hebb's law. Hebb's law is the main principle of neuroplasticity. It states: 'neurons that fire together wire together' (Doidge 2007, p. 63). When two neurons repeatedly simultaneously fire or one fires to set off another, chemical changes happen that forge stronger connections between those two neurons. The chemical changes happen where the neurons meet at the synapse. The synapse is the 'junction between one neuron (brain cell) and another, across which nerve impulses travel' (PositScience Companion Guide 2005–2007, p. 82).

Interaction involves both facilitation (helping – speeding up) and inhibition (hindering – slowing down). Being dynamic the process translates into behaviour that can be modulated and re-modulated and re-modulated – constantly changing – so if the sensory pathway is used it develops and strengthens and becomes more sophisticated – if it is not used it shrinks/fades/disappears. So to sum up, our brains change according to the stimulation we process – process being the operative word. These anatomical and physiological changes continue throughout the life of the individual.

Our senses are everything

All human experience depends on our ability to use our senses. Everything we do is informed by our senses. Each of our senses provides different types of information, which when processed, collectively bestows us with a tremendously rich, multidimensional understanding of what it means to be a human being. Naturally the more multisensory the experience, the more sophisticated our understanding is likely to become.

Multisensory stimulation not only makes it possible for us to survive but it also enables us to thrive in the environment in which we live. Furthermore multisensory stimulation plays a vital role in our personal wellbeing. The reverse is also accurate. Without multisensory stimulation we are cut off from ourselves and from the outside world. We are starved of our own humanity. This is because sensory stimulation is the source of all human meaning and enjoyment – our purpose and our rewards. Our relationship with our senses is what makes life worth living. Over time the way we perceive sensory stimulation becomes our own perception of our selves. Multisensory stimulation therefore supplies the very building blocks of who we are and who we become.

In many ways our access to this stimulation is just taken for granted. This is because mostly our bodies automatically ensure we get the sensory stimulation we require for personal comfort, development, growth, happiness and ongoing maintenance. Furthermore our brains seem to effortlessly become aware of, recognise and interpret these stimuli. Just being in the world is usually enough to stimulate multisensory engagement with self, objects, other people and events. Because of our innate genetic programming as babies we simply learn to use our senses by using them and this is a lifelong process.

For most people this is a spontaneous, innate process but not always. Some, for example those with sense impairments, sensory processing difficulties or brain damage, may not have such a positive and dependable relationship with their senses. For them sense experiences may not even register and if they do, they may lack meaning, be profoundly problematic, unpleasant or even frightening.

Thinking about the senses as multisensory rather than as a disparate set of single yet isolated senses in competition with each other is a significant departure from the historical suppositions embedded in our culture and language. In his *A history of the senses: from antiquity to cyberspace* Jütte (2005, p. 54) observed that the 'number of the senses . . . [was] set firmly at five both in the Western tradition and in early Indian and Chinese culture'. Apparently Aristotle (born around BC 348) not only identified five separate senses, he also pronounced their order of importance as being sight, hearing, smell, taste and touch. Even though nowadays these early notions of the senses are widely acknowledged as social constructs, it is important to be aware of how they have subtly and not so subtly influenced the way people generally think about the senses.

According to Korsmeyer (1998), over the centuries a philosophical argument transpired where sight and hearing were signified as superior because they were thought to be more capable of accessing information from a distance. This apparently made such sense information more objective. However, as taste and touch access information from close proximity, so the argument goes, this made such information more subjective, self-indulgent and inferior.

In due course a binary opposition emerged with vision and hearing occupying positions of dominance, while taste and touch were determined to be more low-grade. A style of communication evolved where visual metaphors are commonly employed to evoke positions of power and authority. For example a politician being interviewed might begin a statement with 'look' or 'see here', expressions that subtly privilege the power of vision. Conversely Hull (2000) reminds us that in the Bible blindness is often associated with negative concepts such as sinful behaviour or not believing in God. Hull goes on to argue that the privileging of a particular sense leads to the privileging of people who have that sense at the expense of those who do not.

Recent scientific evidence now refutes Aristotle's pronouncement. Rather than working in competition with each other, our senses naturally operate at their most efficient in cooperation with one another:

> There can be no doubt that our senses are designed to function in concert and that our brains are organized to use the information they derive from their various sensory channels cooperatively in order to enhance the probability that objects and events will be detected rapidly, identified correctly, and responded to appropriately. Thus, even those experiences that at first may appear to be modality specific are most likely to have been influenced by activity in other sensory modalities, despite our lack of awareness of such interactions.
>
> (Calvert *et al.* 2004, p. xi)

As alluded to previously, nowadays there is debate as to precisely how many different senses we have. For example some argue that vision itself may constitute a combination of discrete senses: one to discern shape, one to discern colour, one to discern three dimensions. Touch can be subdivided into four discrete senses: temperature, vibration, pain and pressure.

However many there are, orchestration of all our senses is crucial. This is so information we detect about our internal selves and our external environment is processed swiftly and accurately, thereby setting us up to make the most appropriate response possible to ensure safety, security, nourishment, reproduction and overall wellbeing. Our brain, the senses and multisensory stimulation all work together. Multisensory stimulation is essential for neuroplasticity to occur.

Modern research indicates that the more multisensory the stimulation, the more likely it will be perceived in more accurate, valid and dependable ways. This is a tremendously important point, especially when working with people who are experiencing difficulties with their senses, perception and sensory processing, because it implies that a more holistic approach may provide a key strategy to help them overcome their difficulties.

Sensory deprivation

A litany of unpleasant scientific research reports exists in the literature detailing the insidious negative effects of sensory deprivation on animals and insects and how this lack of stimulation causes abnormal behaviour. Sadly many examples also abound that catalogue the extreme negative effects of sensory deprivation on humans, particularly children. Prolonged sensory deprivation in young children evidently results in severe disturbances in physical development, social and emotional functioning, behaviour and communication, learning and even compromises the very survival of the child. For example Joseph (1999, p. 193) in a review of the literature reported that:

> [I]n several well known studies of children raised in foundling homes during the early 1900s, when the need for emotional contact was not well recognized, morbidity rates for children less than 1 year of age was generally over 70%. Of 10,272 children admitted to the Dublin Foundling home during a single 25 year period, only 45 survived. Children who survive an infancy spent in institutions where mothering and contact comfort were minimized, display low intelligence, extreme passivity, apathy, severe attentional deficits, pathological shyness, and exceedingly bizarre social behavior.

An oft-cited study by Spitz (1945) gives a strikingly similar account. This study detailed how over 100 children reared in a foundling home with minimal stimulation spent their time obsessively engaged in strange self-stimulatory behaviours and strenuously blocking all adult attempts to interact with them by incessant crying.

I have had personal experience of this phenomenon. It occurred when I started working with an eight-month-old baby girl whom I will call Janine. Janine was both deaf and blind. She was the only child of young parents who lived a long way away from their own parents. I was briefed that Janine had been left to spend most of her time unstimulated and alone in her cot. Her mum said she 'was no trouble at all' and she 'preferred to be left alone'. So Janine had slept often more than twenty hours a day.

Neither mum nor dad had yet bonded with Janine. She was not breastfed. Before coming home from hospital Janine had been in a humidicrib and was already sleeping for long periods of time. By the time she came home, she did not seem to like being handled. When her parents looked at Janine she did not look back so there was no eye contact and when they talked to Janine she did not respond so there was no conversational contact either. Over the ensuing weeks they gave up and let her be, feeding and changing her but little else.

It took me six weeks of visits and working with the parents before I was able to even start to engage with Janine. During those first six weeks every time I tried to pick Janine up she would vehemently scream in protest and nothing I did would dissuade her. It was the same for both her parents. At the time I remember reflecting on Rene Spitz's research and wondering whether Janine's sensory deprivation was simply a result of neglect and lack of know-how, or whether her dual impairments had somehow substantially intensified the deprivation.

As soon as we made our first breakthrough in week six and Janine stopped crying we began a campaign of multisensory stimulation and her resistant behaviour gradually started to abate. Once I was able to demonstrate to the parents that Janine would not protest at being held we purchased a child carrier and the multisensory stimulation began in earnest. The key was convincing mum and dad to use the papoose to keep Janine near them as often as possible, a radical change to their previous behaviour. Fortunately they started to involve Janine in everything they were doing and the changes in Janine's behaviour provided its own reward.

But this type of early intervention does not always happen. Perry and Pollard (1997) published a disturbing picture of two brain scans of three-year-old children, one of a typical child and the other of a child who had been subjected to extreme sensory deprivation. The scan of the child who had been neglected shows a brain with significant cortical atrophy (withering) within a much smaller head. Clearly lack of sensory stimulation through global neglect, deprivations to many different domains, has a substantial effect on the developing brain. Furthermore recent research into neuroplasticity indicates that profound lack of sensory stimulation over an extended period of time has a consequent negative effect on all human brains, no matter what age the person is.

Sometimes sensory deprivation is deliberate and horrific. For example Koluchova (1972, 1976) reported on a pair of identical twin boys from Czechoslovakia. Their mother died soon after their birth so they were placed in social care for about twelve months and then looked after for a further six months by a maternal aunt. During this time their development was normal. When their father, who travelled a lot, remarried, the twins came to live with a cruel step-mother who, for the next five years, kept them in a dark cellar, fed them with meagre scraps and beat them regularly. When discovered the seven-year-old twins were very small, could not speak, had rickets, were afraid of people and were assessed as having severe, permanent, physical and intellectual disabilities.

Surprisingly the twins made an unanticipated recovery. They were enrolled in a special school for children with profound learning disabilities and adopted by a particularly proactive woman who oversaw a programme of stimulation and education. By age fourteen the boys had caught up with their same-age peers and were assessed as being within the normal range both scholastically and emotionally. They went on live stable productive lives. Both married, had children of their own and held down responsible jobs.

When this story was published it sent shock waves around the medical, psychology and education worlds because it radically challenged the assumption of the brain's immutability. Prior to this time emphasis had been placed on the idea of essential critical stages of development within a specific timeframe. This idea was challenged by the fact that these two boys were able to catch up to their same-age peers. The human brain has an amazing ability of self-repair, providing the right conditions for this repair are provided. Subsequent literature started to be much more cautious with the way it discussed critical stages of development.

Early sensory stimulation approaches

Sensory deprivation not only occurs from abuse or neglect, it is also caused by severe sense impairment and learning disabilities. Because of this our society has a moral responsibility to try to minimise sensory deprivation in children and adults with sense impairment and learning disabilities. Despite the horror stories associated with sensory deprivation there are examples where practitioners have tried to provide sensory stimulation to people who might otherwise be sensorially deprived. For example Cleland and Clark (1966, p. 213), two psychologists who worked in the USA, developed a 'sensory cafeteria' for people with intellectual disability who lived in an institution to reduce their abnormal behaviour.

A few years later, in the early 1970s, Hulsegge and Verheul created a similar sensory approach to keep the 440 participants with intellectual and multiple disabilities at the De Hartenberg Centre in the Netherlands gainfully occupied. Hulsegge and Verheul called their areas for sensory stimulation a Snoezelen, a word they created by combining the Dutch words: '"snuffelin" = to sniff, to snuffle and "doezelen" = to doze, to snooze' (Verheul 2007, p. 8).

As the story goes, one evening after work Ad Verheul and Jan Hulsegge had a social get together, where they started talking about what a pity it was their participants never got to experience simple social pleasures such as going to the pub. They discussed how life for their participants was always the same, always predictable, with very little change, very little to occupy them. They wondered whether there was anything they could do about it. After more discussion they decided to conduct an experiment, so they went back to the centre and found a participant who was just sitting in a wheelchair doing nothing, seemingly completely disengaged. They wheeled him out into the cool evening air for a few minutes, then wheeled him back inside. His reaction was one of sheer delight. He started laughing and interacting in ways that were surprising – out of character. Something had happened that caught his attention – he became engaged.

Inside the building was always kept at a constant temperature, whereas outside it was cool. Ad and Jan believed that it was the change in temperature that made the difference. This inspired Ad and Jan and other staff at the centre to design a series of rooms to create a 'dream atmosphere', which provided 'stimuli for every sense' (Verheul 2007, p. 16), and was very different to their day-to-day life in the institution. They told their story in a book entitled *Snoezelen another world: a practical book of sensory experience environments for the mentally handicapped* (Hulsegge and Verheul 1986).

Once their book was published, similar rooms for children and adults with sensory and learning disabilities were constructed in different locations throughout Europe and around the world. Within a fairly short period of time the word Snoezelen® had became a registered trademark for the British company ROMPA, so new terms and approaches to multisensory stimulation began to appear such as multisensory environments, controlled multisensory environments, multisensory rooms, sensory trolleys and sensory theatre to name but a few.

Multisensory stimulation refers to information that simultaneously appeals to more than one set of sense nerve receptors. It is this synchronized alliance of the senses that creates entirely new abilities or ways of gaining information about the world that would not be possible through one sense organ alone. The key message is that the more multisensory the stimulation, the more likely the information will be perceived in accurate, valid and dependable ways. The idea of us using a particular sense in isolation is somewhat illusory. We are multisensory beings – our senses work in concert with each other, even when we think they are operating in seclusion. Therefore using multisensory stimulation to help children and adults with sensory and learning disabilities is a most natural, logical and optimistic approach.

Sense organs and sensory processing

Introduction

In Chapter 2 we will explore the senses in greater detail and along the way we will start to learn more about multisensory stimulation. We begin with an introduction to each of the major sense organs and examine how and why particular senses work together. For example one sense may provide a foundation upon which another sense builds or two senses may work together to create a new form of perception. We then start to think about the basic concepts behind sensory processing. In particular we focus on the idea of sensory threshold, that is the need for the sense stimulus to be powerful enough for it to be detected, recognised and differentiated so that it can be compared with other sense stimuli.

Sense organs

Information about the inside and outside world reaches the CNS via a variety of sense receptors. A collection of similar types of sense receptors embedded in non-neuronal tissue is called a sense organ. These sense receptors within the sense organ can be regarded as operating collectively to achieve a common task.

We have hundreds of millions of sense receptors of many different types. Some are simple nerve endings and some are specialised cells. They are all transducers that convert energy in the environment into electrical activity in nerves. Before they can respond, sense receptors require an adequate stimulus, in other words the type of stimulus must match the transduction capability of the receptor. Humans have at least six receptor types, perhaps more. They are:

1   Chemoreceptors respond to chemical stimuli (e.g. smell, taste).
2   Mechanoreceptors respond to mechanical stress or strain to detect changes in pressure, position or acceleration (e.g. stretch, touch, hearing, equilibrium).
3   Nocireceptors respond to tissue damage (leads to pain perception).
4   Photoreceptors respond to light (e.g. vision).
5   Proprioreceptors respond to position (e.g. proprioception).
6   Thermoreceptors respond to temperature (e.g. touch).

On the stimulus reaching a particular threshold an individual receptor depolarises, sending an action potential along its associated nerve. The threshold for each sense receptor within the sense organ is different for each receptor. As the barrage of action potentials generated by the stimulus is relayed via neurones, via synapses to the spinal cord and brain, integration occurs. The integration gives information as to the stimulus intensity, location and duration.

Sensory receptors can be divided into two broad classes: interoception and exteroception. These receptors combine to inform the individual where self ends, where the environment begins and how the two interrelate. The sense organs described in this chapter are explored from inside out, that is interoception then exteroception as this order seems to more closely resemble the way the senses emerge in the developing organism.

Interoception (from the Latin *internus* 'inside') describes senses that access stimuli from inside the body. It encompasses proprioception, the vestibular sense, and any other sense receptor stimulated from within the body. This includes sensory receptors in the lungs for breathing, in the stomach to indicate thirst, hunger or discomfort and in the bladder and rectum to signal emptying.

Proprioception (from the Latin *proprius* 'own' and *capere* 'to take') and kinesthesia (from the Greek *kinein* 'to move', *aisthesis* 'perception') are overlapping concepts that refer to the sensations of position, tension and movement of body parts whether stationary or in flux. For simplicity I will use the term 'proprioception' throughout the remainder of this book.

Proprioceptors access stimuli that describe the current state of our body in relation to gravity. Proprioception tells us where we are located in space. The vestibular sense determines our ability to perceive rotary acceleration, keep our head in position (essential for vision) and to maintain an upright posture in relation to the external environment.

Roger Sperry, 1981 Nobel-prize recipient for physiology or medicine, is attributed to have estimated that more than 90 per cent of the brain's energy goes into posture alone. If this is the case then interoception is much more important than is generally acknowledged, particularly in the field of education. Because these senses collectively provide an intrinsic feedback mechanism that enables the individual to monitor and maintain their own stability relative to the external environment, they are closely connected with motor development and the maintenance of motor skills across the life span. Furthermore interoception plays a vital role in providing a foundational base from which exteroception may occur.

Exteroception (from the Latin *externus* 'outside') describes senses that access stimuli from outside the body. For these senses to be able to access this information, however, they need to have a context and this context comes from proprioception and the vestibular sense. The senses of exteroception are therefore already multisensory in nature because they work in conjunction with the senses of interoception. The senses of exteroception are sorted into: exteroception (near), that is senses that inform the person about their immediate world, such as taste, smell, touch and the cutaneous senses (pressure, pain and temperature), and exteroception (distant), that is senses that, in addition to providing information about the immediate world, also access more distant information, such as hearing and vision.

The senses of exteroception provide the individual with the large majority of information that goes into informing the conscious self. As a consequence, we are especially aware of these senses. However the nervous system largely keeps the information provided by interoception at an unconscious level. That explains why we tend to think of the senses of exteroception as being of far greater importance.

The senses of interoception

Close your eyes and rest your arms by your side. Keep your eyes closed and raise the index finger on your right hand to touch your nose. Now try the same action with your left hand index finger. To execute this activity you need to use interoception.

Proprioceptors in the muscles and tendons ultimately provide the individual with sensations of position, tension and movement of body parts. The muscle spindle is a proprioceptor that provides information about changes in muscle length, and the Golgi tendon organ provides information about changes in muscle tension.

Muscle spindles are found throughout the body of each muscle, parallel with the muscle fibres. The Golgi tendon organs are in series with the muscle fibres, in the tendons that attach muscle to bone. Together they respond to three types of changes in muscle force, a passive change when the muscle is pulled (as in massage), and two active changes: isometric and isotonic contractions. These two active changes involve muscular contraction against resistance however, with isometric the length of the muscle remains constant while the tension changes, and with isotonic the tension remains constant while the length changes.

Muscle spindles have both motor and sensory components. They provide and receive information regarding changes in muscle length and muscle force to maintain a two-way communication with the CNS. In this way, through integration, purposeful movement is achieved.

Muscle spindles are thought to play a particularly vital role in sensorimotor development. Sensorimotor development occurs when the infant starts to co-ordinate sensory experiences with motor activity. For example touching your nose with your index finger is clearly a sensorimotor activity. In addition to involving the senses of interoception, the arm must actually move the finger to the nose, so the motor is involved.

Piaget (1928) described the sensorimotor as the first stage in cognitive development. It typically progresses from birth through to age two. During the first six weeks of life the baby gradually develops increased control over basic reflexes such as sucking and grasping. This makes them more voluntary and in the process changes them in qualitative ways. For example the palmer grasp becomes an intentional hand movement, which can grasp at will. This initiates a series of development that eventually makes it possible for someone to close their eyes and touch their nose.

The vestibular sense receptors are located in the semi-circular canals, saccules and utricles of the inner ear. They consist of hair cells that bend when the fluid in which they are bathed (perilimph) moves. The three semi-circular canals in both the left and right inner ears are positioned at right angles to each other so as to provide maximum information about the movement. The two sets engage in a push–pull action with their corresponding set. As one set is stimulated (facilitated), the other set is inhibited, thereby providing greater detail and precision regarding acceleration/de-acceleration. The semi-circular canals particularly respond to rotary acceleration. The saccules and utricles are similar but particularly respond to linear acceleration. The vestibular system helps in coordination of the body during running, walking and all movements of the head.

The senses of exteroception

Even though the senses of exteroception are divided into two groups, namely near and distant, this division is not completely airtight. There is considerable blurring of boundaries. For example, as we will discover, the cutaneous senses provide information about both the internal and external worlds, and smell may accesses information from a considerable distance as well as up close.

Taste and smell both belong to the chemical sensing system called chemosensation. In addition to taste and smell, a third chemical sense located in the moist surfaces of the eyes, nose, mouth and throat, identifies sensations such as the 'stinging' feeling associated with ammonia, the 'coolness' of menthol and the 'hot sensation' of chilli.

Taste (gustation), sometimes called the gatekeeper to the body, provides us with information about substances in solutions, whereas smell (olfaction) provides us with information about substances in gaseous form. Gustatory receptors (taste buds) are predominately found in the mouth, whereas olfactory receptors originate in the nasal passages. As is the case for the majority of sensory systems both gustatory and olfactory receptors are associated with tiny hairs.

Most taste buds are on the tongue, although they are also located in other parts of the mouth, throat and even in the lungs (Deshpande *et al.* 2010). Research now refutes the idea of a tongue map, with taste receptors now thought to spread relatively evenly around the whole tongue. The four main types of taste receptors are sweet (sugars), salt, sour (acid) and bitter (alkaloids). Umami, a fifth type, refers to the ability to recognise a somewhat brothy, meaty taste sensation from glutamate. Olfactory receptors (about 40 million of them) are located at the base of the bridge of the nose in a match head size olfactory bulb. These receptors enable a person to be able to distinguish up to 10,000 odours.

Chemosensation makes it possible for us to enjoy the delights of life, such as the smell of flowers or the flavours of food and drink. It also plays an essential role in warning us of impending danger, such as fire or poisons. Babies from a very early age can identify their mother through smell (especially if she is breast feeding). Smells signal the familiar: people, places and objects. They therefore play an important role in the development of memory. Furthermore chemosensation becomes a strong motivator in the development and refining of eating and drinking skills, such as sucking, chewing and swallowing. These activities encourage good muscle tone, a prerequisite for speech.

Taste and smell are often confused because taste combines with other sensations to form a common chemical sense alliance called flavour. In addition to taste flavour consists of temperature, texture and especially smell. Flavour is important for identifying and recognising what we consume. The tongue houses highly sensitive touch sensors, which provide considerable information about whatever is in the mouth, particularly texture. Smell takes place primarily through inhalation whereas flavour happens primarily through exhalation.

Sound also influences the perceived flavour experience. Next time you eat a potato crisp notice how much more enjoyable it is when it is fresh and crunchy compared to consuming it once it has become soft after exposure to the air. As a further indulgence quickly devour a very cold drink and notice the resulting brain freeze. This is because thermoreceptors down your digestive tract have provided your brain with an abundant amount of information regarding its sub-zero temperature.

Smell fades after a person has been exposed to it for a period of time. Olfactory fatigue occurs because the person has become accustomed to that smell. Other senses that also go through a process of fatigue include taste, touch, vision and hearing. The first taste is the sharpest, most intense. Then if we continue to eat the same thing, over time the taste subsides. As discussed in Chapter 1 people only notice sense experiences that are different. If a person lives in an unchanging environment then that person notices less and less over time. Remember Janine the eight-month-old-girl who was deaf and blind. She not only experienced extreme sensory fatigue, she vehemently objected to any form of change.

The tactual and cutaneous senses, otherwise known as the somatic senses or the somatosensory system (from Greek *soma* 'body'), comprise touch (tactition), pressure, temperature and pain. These senses are found in the skin covering the entire human body, which makes them tremendously important to our wellbeing.

A point-to-point map of the body to corresponding parts of the brain, called the cortical homunculus, provides a general idea as to which locations in the brain oversee particular body parts and functions. This cortical map, however, is not immutable. After brain damage or trauma to particular body parts shifts may occur. The term 'tactile' refers to passive touch, such as the sensation a cap on your head gives you when you are wearing it. The touch experience of wearing clothing undergoes a fairly rapid fatigue meaning that most of the time we are hardly aware of its feel. Active touch or haptic (from Greek *haptein* 'touch') perception involves the alliance of somatosensory perception and proprioception as well as the activation of the motor and the sensorimotor. Haptic perception involves the interface between the person's body and their immediate outside world. It plays a key role in the recognition of objects by touch. Haptic technolology, which involves extended physiological proprioception, can range from simple devices such as a white cane used by people who are blind to get around independently, through to complicated robotic surgery conducted through virtual reality systems.

Functional touch is any use of touch that adds to the person's experience, enjoyment and learning about the world. Touch is enormously important in human activity. It is an essential component in motor activities. Touch enables us to learn how to manipulate and shape of the world. It involves the discrimination of: textures (rough to smooth); density (hard to soft); state (gas to fluid to solid); surface to depth (palpation); size (small to large); temperature (hot to cold); vibration (static to gentle to vigorous); shape (circle, square). Tactual exploration is a sequential process where one part is joined to other parts to provide an overall impression of the whole. This means that a large number of sophisticated skills are involved, including the higher order functions of memory, spatial ability, gross and fine motor development and scanning. Research indicates that touch, in addition to wellbeing, is essential for physical, emotional and intellectual development. This point was highlighted in Chapter 1 in the section on sensory deprivation.

Hearing is similar to touch in so far as it also uses mechanoreceptors to detect the movement of molecules. The ability to perceive sound primarily occurs within the auditory system although some sound vibrations can be detected through other body parts such as our bones. The auditory system consists of two ears each comprising three parts: outer ear, middle ear and inner ear.

Sounds have two parameters, frequency (pitch) measured in Hertz (Hz) and intensity (loudness) measured in decibels (dB). One Hertz is one cycle (sound wave) per second. The word sonic is used to describe the frequencies the human ear can detect. These range from about 20 Hz (very low pitch) to 20,000 Hz (very high pitch), but dogs can hear even higher frequencies (referred to as ultrasonic) and elephants can hear even lower frequencies (referred to as infrasonic). The pressure of the sound wave flowing through air is measured in decibels. Humans can hear sounds from 0 dB (the lower volume limit of audible sound) through to 120 dB, the pain threshold. Sounds beyond this volume damage the eardrum. Being logarithmic 120 dB is 1,000,000,000,000 times louder than 0 dB.

The pinna (folds of cartilage surrounding the ear canal) of the outer ear access sound waves and reflect them along the trumpet shaped ear canal towards the eardrum (tympanic membrane). The eardrum, which is the entrance to the middle ear, converts pressure into amplitude. Within the middle ear the newly converted sound waves travel through an air filled cavity along the ossicles – three of the smallest bones in the body. Named because of their shape these bones are the malleus (hammer), incus (anvil) and, the smallest of the three, the stapes (stirrup). The sound then travels through the oval window, the entrance to the inner ear. The fluid filled inner ear is where sound waves are converted into nerve impulses by the hair cells in the cochlea for transmission to the auditory cortex.

Auditory perception involves the two ears working together as a team. For example jointly the two ears provide valuable information about the source of the sound. In a procedure similar to the interchange between the two sets of semi-circular canals, the closer ear detects the sound earlier than the more distant one, thereby enabling location determination.

Vision is the most enormously rich sense we have, and it accounts for the majority of our conscious perceptions. We can see objects very close up and in the night sky we can also see objects hundreds of millions of kilometres away. The two eyes are each housed inside the bony bowls of the skull, cushioned by fatty layers, and controlled by a set of six muscles. These enable the eye to move through a vast field of vision, almost 100 degrees from top to bottom and 180 degrees from side to side. Further protection is afforded the eyes by the eyelids that can be closed to form an airtight and waterproof shield, and opened at will to allow light to enter into the eye. The white outer surface of the eye, the sclera, has a transparent centre called the cornea. The sclera provides nourishment to the eye and keeps out all non-essential light, thereby optimising visual functioning.

A transparent membrane the conjunctiva, which covers the cornea, is kept moist by oily tears secreted by the lacrimal gland, and uniformly spread over the eye's surface by regular blinking. Light from an external source enters the eye through the lens and the cornea and then passes through the pupil, an aperture formed by the iris, a pigmented muscle that expands and contracts to regulate the amount of available light entering the base of the eye. This action is called the papillary light reflex and happens automatically in response to the external intensity of the light.

Light that enters the eye is bent by the cornea and the lens. It subsequently travels through vitreous humour, a transparent jelly like fluid, to eventually hit the retina at the back of the eye as an inverted image. Focusing is achieved by ciliary muscle action, which changes the shape of the lens, more round for near vision and more oval for distant. Accommodation occurs when focus is maintained over time. Accommodative and fusional vergence occurs when the eyes maintain focus at one distance, then quickly change to accurately focus at a different distance. When the two eyes are aimed exactly at the same point at the same time this is called near point of convergence. Near point of convergence plays a valuable role in stereopsis, which leads to the perception of depth.

The retina consists of about 130 million photoreceptors, which are divided into two types, rods and cones. The rods are located more at the periphery of the retina whereas cones are found more in the centre. Rods enable the eyes to see in dim light and provide information about shape. The three kinds of cones (short blue, middle green and long red) help us distinguish colour in up to 10 million shades, but function best in strong light. As candlepower diminishes the eyes' ability to discern, colour similarly reduces.

An example of how exteroception is predicated on interoception is the way vision depends on the vestibular system to provide a basis for perception of the world in three dimensions. The vestibular system ensures that head movements are compensated for so that images on the retina are stabilised.

Sensory processing

Previously we described a sense as any faculty that accesses stimuli from inside or outside the body with perception the act of becoming aware of, recognising and interpreting these stimuli. Due to the difficulty involved in trying to distinguish between sense and perception, sensory processing was introduced as an umbrella term to account for both and to focus on the interface where a sense ends and perception begins. Individual sense receptors have an all-or-none response, that is they either fire or they do not. However, whether a stimulus is perceived or not, and how it is perceived, depends on higher order processing beyond the sense organ.

It is important to differentiate between sensation and perception. The clarity of information accessed by the sense organ is called sense acuity. For example 20/20 vision means a person can clearly discern a visual image that is 20 metres away from a distance of 20 metres. A person with vision impairment, however, might only be able to see the same image from one metre so we call that level of visual acuity 1/20 vision. We also talk about visual acuity for both close (near visual acuity) and distance (distance visual acuity). A person with a near visual acuity problem may need to bring an object closer to the eye to be able to see it. This helps to demonstrate how the sense and the brain work together to achieve a better result.

Each sense organ has a sense acuity, which is that sense organ's actual physical ability to clearly and sharply receive the sense information. For example we measure hearing in terms of frequency (pitch) and volume. An audiogram is used to chart whether the person has average hearing along frequency and volume axes, or whether the person has some hearing loss. Acuity needs are addressed with prosthetic devices such as magnifying glasses and hearing aids. The brain is wholly dependent on the quality of the initial stimulus collected.

Perception entails the brain making comparisons with other information already stored in the brain, referring to information that was gathered from past experiences. Perception therefore involves memory and many other cognitive abilities. It is therefore vital to recognise that sense acuity is different to perception. A person might have good visual acuity but poor visual processing ability, whereas another person may have poor visual acuity but good visual processing ability. On the one hand, a person with good visual acuity but poor visual processing ability may see things but just not understand the significance of what is being observed. On the other hand, a person with poor visual acuity and good visual processing ability may see very little but have extremely sophisticated understanding regarding what is being observed.

Sensory thresholds

In Chapter 1 I said a simple sensory stimulus, if powerful enough, triggers a nerve receptor, which can in turn set in motion a cascade of neural electrical impulses. I now want to look more closely at this idea of 'if powerful enough'. If powerful enough refers to the idea of a threshold. A threshold is defined as a boundary, the point that must be exceeded to produce a given effect or result or response. With sensory processing, which is essentially integrative in nature, three different thresholds are relevant. These are: detection threshold, recognition threshold and differential threshold.

The detection threshold is the minimum stimulus required for it to be detected by a human sense organ. For example a sound must reach a certain volume and frequency for it to be detected by the human ear. In humans this is usually above 20 Hertz and 0 decibels although it may be considerably higher if the person has a hearing impairment, or a sensory processing disorder. Some animals such as elephants can detect lower frequencies and softer sounds, such as the approach of a tsunami. We might not hear a sound, but that does not mean the environment is soundless. It just means the sounds were not powerful enough to go over our particular sound detection threshold.

The same could be said about vision. A person with regular vision can see only red to violet in the visible spectrum, but not infrared or ultraviolet (because these are outside the baseline thresholds). Infrared has a longer wavelength than the visible spectrum but some animals such as vampire bats can use infrared to locate food. Likewise ultraviolet has a shorter wavelength than the visible spectrum yet parrots see ultraviolet plumage (thought to play a role in mating) and koalas use it to locate eucalyptus trees way off in the distance.

Although there is a normal range, all thresholds are different for each person and they change across time and circumstance. I use the term detection threshold in preference to absolute and terminal thresholds, the terms used in the literature. This is because the terms absolute and terminal thresholds suggest they are fixed, whereas at an individual level thresholds change with use, experience, ability, age, context and a range of other variables. That is, unless the person is missing that particular sense altogether, such as being totally blind because of damage to the eye, in which case the threshold would not be relevant. A powerful way to lower a threshold is by expectation. For instance if you are expecting a particular sound then even if it is very soft the ear may just be able to make it out, whereas if you are otherwise occupied and not expecting the sound it could easily be missed. A second reason for using the term detection threshold is to emphasise that we are focusing on a particular individual's threshold, not a threshold for the population in general.

The recognition threshold is the level of stimulus required for the person to both detect and recognise it. This is a higher level of processing than just detection. For example, have you ever thought you could smell smoke and rushed outside to check whether you were accurate? You did this by searching for a stronger sense signal, to allow you to confirm your suspicions. You needed a stronger sense signal to be able to go beyond detection and actually recognise it.

It is important to make a distinction between the detection and recognition threshold because some children and adults might be able to detect a sense stimulus but they cannot recognise it. They do not have the sense stimuli readily accessible in their memory bank to be able to make a match.

Memory is the process of being able to recall a stimulus. There are three key types of memory, namely: short-term memory (STM), long-term memory (LTM) and working memory. STM only lasts for seconds and is the initial laying-down of the neural electrical cascade. Repetition, rehearsal and meaningful association change STM into LTM. As LTM is subject to fading in the natural forgetting process, many recalls/retrievals are needed for LTM to persist.

Working memory is the ability to hold and manipulate information in the mind over short periods of time. It is a kind of mental workspace used to store important information in the course of our everyday lives. A good example of an activity that uses working memory is mental arithmetic. Plainly people with dementia are susceptible to experiencing problems in this area. Another group of people who may experience problems are those with autism, especially the young child.

According to Williams *et al.* (2006) people with autism have two particular problems with working memory:

1   They have a poor working memory for spatial information.
2   They do not have an automatic cross talk process between reasoning and memory systems that tells their brain what is most important to notice and how to organise it.

This is why some people with autism use self-talk as a way of monitoring their own behaviour. The information needs to come out in the form of speech and then be reprocessed through listening.

So how is this information about autism relevant to thresholds? Well, it is particularly relevant for the differential threshold. Stimulus that has got over the differential threshold can be analysed for perceived change, for example hearing whether a sound is getting louder or softer, higher or lower, faster or slower. To be able to notice a difference the person must be able to compare and contrast recognised stimuli. This requires a STM, a LTM and a working memory. Processing differential thresholds is a prerequisite of language development.

Donna Williams (1998) in her book *Autism and sensing: the unlost instinct* insightfully explained what was happening to her. 'Nothing could shock me because no interpretation was happening, no judgment and no thought. I appeared to stare into space and stare through things.' She made the same observation regarding her hearing:

> I could hear but had no need to listen and appeared to be deaf (and was tested for deafness at the age of two and again at the age of nine). In response to sudden loud noises, there was no response, not because I was deaf, for I could certainly hear sound and perhaps even more sound and more clearly than most people, but because I had no capacity to process sound, to interpret it and make the normally instinctual physical connections to respond to it.
>
> (Williams 1998, p. 53)

The same kinds of sensory processing problems could be occurring for people with dementia.

Chapter 3

Pleasure, happiness and Predictive Coding

Introduction

In Chapter 1 we learnt about neuroplasticity and how our brains change according to the stimulation we process, with process being the operative word. If the sensory pathway is used, it strengthens and develops but if it is not used it shrinks/fades/disappears. I argued that using multisensory stimulation to help children and adults with sensory and learning disabilities is the most natural, logical and optimistic approach because the right kind of multisensory stimulation for each individual has the potential to strengthen the sensory pathways and promote personal wellbeing. The alternative, leaving people to be perpetually trapped in environments where little or no stimulation is being processed, is difficult to justify.

In Chapter 2 we started to think more about what is the right kind of multisensory stimulation particularly for the senses of exteroception. Even though a sense organ may have the sense acuity to access a particular type of stimulation, the person will not engage with that stimulation unless it is powerful enough to capture their attention. The stimulation has to be supraliminal (i.e. above the threshold, as opposed to subliminal, i.e. below the threshold). Stimulation at the detection threshold, however, only results in mere detection. Higher levels of stimulation experience and expertise are required to get over the recognition threshold where stimulation is identified, and even greater levels of stimulation experience and expertise are necessary to go beyond the differential threshold where stimulation is processed in comparative and more meaningful ways.

Individuals use their senses to purposively engage with sensory stimulation, objects, people and events. The level of engagement is determined by the person's sensory processing ability. But it is more complicated than just processing ability. This is because there is an affective component as well.

People who can detect stimulation but not identify it, or differentiate it, have less affective involvement with the stimulation because it is less meaningful. As sensory processing becomes more sophisticated so too does the ability to remain engaged, and to have an emotional attachment to the sense experience. In short the meaningfulness generated by better engagement in turn generates pleasure in the engagement and vice versa.

Down time

Recently I stayed in a pretty village that contained a collection of stylish modern units inhabited by adults with sensory and learning disabilities. Each adult lived independently in his or her own home. The front of every residence consisted of a large glass window that looked out across well-manicured lawns and gardens onto the street. It was quite an idyllic spot.

As I took an evening stroll around the village, however, I gradually became aware that through every window I could see a person sitting motionless on a chair. It was like the inhabitants had all closed down for the time being, not actively using their senses. I knew that the carers had dutifully ensured their participants were properly bathed, fed and made comfortable and so I surmised that I was witnessing a daily procedure where all the inhabitants were left to have some down time. Except down time for them, in practice, meant doing nothing.

As I walked around this village I wondered how many other such people all over the world spend large amounts of time sensorily disengaged, a state they may only come out of when someone else intervenes. These people, when left to their own devices, cease to engage with the outside world. They simply do not have the momentum to self-engage with the outside world.

To be effective, the person who does intervene, to get such a person to start using their senses, would need to have the skills to get their participant engaged, the time and inclination to want to make it happen, and the perseverance to ensure the engagement was maintained over time. However the greater the intensity and duration of the sensory deprivation experienced by the participant, the more challenging the task would be to re-engage the participant.

While I was in the village I also reflected on an earlier visit to an aged care facility, where people with dementia were similarly having down time. I remembered the residents in the aged care facility looked very much like those people in the village. When a person is not purposively using their senses, he or she takes on an unmistakable appearance. Despite many institutions being disbanded and much greater emphasis now being placed on inclusion, far too many people still experience significant periods of sensory deprivation. These people are not independently engaged in accessing any meaningful sense information.

As we learnt in Chapters 1 and 2, the more time one spends closed off from the world the more vulnerable that person becomes to experiencing even greater levels of sensory deprivation. The sensory deprivation then results in severe disturbances in physical development, social and emotional functioning, behaviour and communication. Paradoxically when these disturbances arise, rather than giving the person abundant amounts of the right kinds of multisensory stimulation, often the person is simply prescribed a sedative or anti-anxiety medication. This might hide the symptoms but it often exacerbates the sensory deprivation. So what constitutes the right kinds of multisensory stimulation?

It all starts with success

I recall, many, many years ago talking to an ophthalmologist about John, one of my students with visual impairment and learning disabilities who was about ten years old at the time. I wanted to know what I could do to overcome the problem of him refusing to wear his glasses. The ophthalmologist said:

> John is only going to keep his glasses on if he gets sufficient visual reward from the experience. He refuses to wear his glasses because he's not getting enough return for effort. There is too much frustration and not enough success.

This conversation changed the way I interacted with John. Previously I had been demanding compliance, telling him what to do. I insisted: 'John, don't take your glasses off. Put your glasses back on.' I gave him pragmatic reasons to justify my demands: 'You need your glasses for the next activity.' Up until then I had not been considering the situation from John's perspective. I simply thought he has glasses so he should wear them, and it is my job to make him do so.

After talking to the ophthalmologist I had an entirely different strategy at my disposal. I could concentrate on what kind of visual reward John was experiencing. I could try to understand his relationship with seeing and help him find more authentic visual rewards – ones that were personally relevant, meaningful and of special value to him. I already knew what John's interests were. He was fascinated with motorbikes. I therefore went to the library and borrowed the best picture books and magazines I could find. I also collected other resources from friends. Pretty soon I had amassed an impressive collection of material on motorbikes.

One day when John was not wearing his glasses I asked if he could help me. I explained I had a poster of a motorbike but I could not work out what make it was. Could he help me? I then showed him my collection of information on motorbikes. John's glasses immediately took on a new currency. Not only did he put them on without my coaxing, he also made use of all the low vision aids he could find in the classroom. Soon he was able to inform me that it was a Moto Guzzi – a 1969 V7 750 Speciale. I then asked John if he could describe the Moto Guzzi logo, which started a new search. From then on every time he came up with an answer, I would ask a new question about motorbikes that required John to make more precise use of his vision, and off he would go to enthusiastically search out the answer. We were on a run. He was learning to use his vision by using it. He was actively involved.

The more I learned about John, his interests, his likes and dislikes, the better I became at designing increasingly more demanding visual learning experiences, where he achieved success on his own terms. It was his success because it was meaningful to him. Over time he became more comfortable about wearing his glasses in the classroom for schoolwork. Out in the playground, though, it was a completely different story. Clearly John had other issues to consider in the playground.

What is success?

At its most basic level success is being able to achieve that which is attempted. Everything we do is either successful or it is not. For example if I decided I wanted to scratch my arm and then did it – that is success. I achieved what I set out to do. If I did not achieve it, I would experience failure. I would feel frustrated.

The key point here is most of us are so used to success we take it for granted. Our lives consist of billions of unrecognized success stories that all flow into one another. Every move we make started with an intention followed by an outcome, which was either a success or a failure. We wake up in the morning, get out of bed, walk towards the bathroom, clean our teeth and so on. We experience success experience upon success experience. It is these success stories that keep up our momentum.

It is important to remind ourselves just how much we take success for granted and to be aware that somewhere along the success–failure continuum is a cut-off point where the success momentum is not sufficiently strong to keep up the flow. The people in the village and those in the aged care facility were experiencing insufficient success and this was inhibiting engagement.

To help illustrate my point about how we take success for granted, try the following activity. First of all close your eyes and write your name. I imagine you found that relatively easy, no problem at all and your signature looks almost identical to the one you usually write. Now close your eyes again and write your name using your non-dominant hand. Did you find that a little more challenging? What if you keep your eyes closed and continue to use your non-dominant hand, but this time sign your name back-to-front and upside down? Perhaps this time you will experience a greater level of failure? Notice how you react. Are you tempted to just give up or are you willing to persevere and keep on trying? The important point here is that, on the one hand, the more success you experience, generally the easier it is to persevere, and the more willing you are to try again. On the other hand, the more failure you experience, generally the harder it is to try again and the less likely you are to even try. So to sum up, success breeds success and failure breeds more failure. The people in the village and those in the aged care facility, when left to themselves, stop engaging with the outside world. They cease to purposively use their senses.

People who achieve success are far better equipped to cope with frustration. The more success they achieve, the more adventurous they are about trying new experiences. The opposite occurs for people who rarely achieve success. They are poorly equipped to cope with frustration. The less success they achieve the more success they need to be willing to try new things. They become afraid of new experiences. Consequently their world shrinks. They learn to be helpless.

Learned helplessness and learned optimism

Seligman (1975) introduced the term 'learned helplessness' to describe a situation where after a series of failures, people and animals alike begin to behave as if the outcome is completely out of their control. They do not equate success with personal effort. It is sad to witness how easily learned helplessness can be induced.

Illustrating how learned helplessness is generated is Seligman and Maier's classic but distressing (1967) experiment on three groups of dogs. Group one dogs were harnessed for a while and then released. Group two dogs were harnessed for the same period of time and given electric shocks but these shocks ceased when the dogs pressed a lever. This meant they had some level of control. Finally the dogs in the third group were harnessed, given electric shocks but they had no way of avoiding the shock because their levers did not work. When all the dogs were released the dogs in groups one and two recovered quickly, whereas the dogs in group three had learned to be helpless. They exhibited symptoms similar to depression. When the group three dogs were subjected to another round of electric shocks the dogs lay down and passively allowed the shocks to be delivered without even trying to escape, even though they could easily have avoided the shocks by jumping over a low partition. People with learned helplessness can behave in equally sad and upsetting ways.

The failure associated with learned helplessness assumes three dimensions (Seligman 1975). First, the failure is felt to be permanent and inevitable. Second, there is a strong connection between the failure and the person who fails, the failure becomes part of the way that the person self-identifies. Third, the failure spreads to all aspects of a person's life. Learned helplessness can be so pervasive that the individual continues to behave in a helpless way in all areas of life, even after opportunities are provided for them to avoid unpleasant and harmful circumstances.

Flannery (2002, p. 345) described learned helplessness as 'the psychological state that results when an individual who is unable to exercise reasonable mastery in one situation incorrectly assumes that he or she is then unable to exercise reasonable control in other situations as well'. Learned helplessness becomes a pervasive self-fulfilling prophesy of defeat. Given the often seemingly insurmountable problems children and adults with sensory and learning disabilities face, it is easy to understand why they are so highly susceptible to experiencing learned helplessness in their daily life.

The opposite of learned helplessness is learned optimism. According to Seligman (1998) people can be immunised against learned helplessness. You do this by providing them with an abundance of positive experiences. Then while the person engages in the activities you increase their awareness of the positive experiences. This can be achieved by asking questions that focus their attention on the positive aspects, for example: 'What are you looking at? You seem to be so content.' You could also use self-talk if the person has a problem with communication: 'You've been watching the bird on the grass. You enjoyed watching that bird so much. Look it's gone under the sprinkler and it's having a shower. You're smiling.'

The next step is to ensure that if a person experiences a failure it is framed as a one-off occurrence, a temporary setback and it is specific to just one area. 'I know you had a little fall but it's very unusual. You hardly ever fall over. You are good at walking and you're always so careful. Perhaps you fell over because it's so dark in here.' Then you can follow up the reframing by providing the person with sufficient scaffolding to help them learn how to translate the failure into success. 'Turn the light on. Let's see if that makes it easier for you. Does that make a difference?'

With multisensory stimulation the practitioner tries to design an environment where the person can experience an abundance of success (positive experiences) and this success is personally relevant and meaningful. Of course being able to design such an experience is a challenge. There are many factors to take into account. The first factor we will consider is pleasure.

What is pleasure?

Pleasure is closely associated with sensory stimulation. Pleasure means deriving enjoyment from a sensory experience. It is a state of being, which involves the gratification of the senses. For most people achieving satisfaction from the senses is a given. It happens automatically. The pleasure derived from the sense experience then provides the motivation for us to continue to use the senses into the future. For example the newborn baby is hungry so the mother offers a satisfying drink of breast milk. Thereafter each time the baby has a feed of breast milk the senses are gratified. The baby can taste the milk. The baby can also smell it. The mother holds the baby in her arms, she gently talks to the baby and exchanges eye contact. Touch is involved. It is a multisensory experience.

People with sensory impairments and learning disabilities, however, may find attaining gratification more difficult. They may experience failure upon failure and stop engaging in a sense activity altogether. For them success does not come easily and using the senses is not automatically a fun experience. For instance the baby might not be able to suck sufficiently well to obtain milk from the breast. The baby might not have sufficient vision to be able to exchange eye contact, to see the mother's smile. Many different things may go wrong with the senses and sensory processing.

Sometimes fixing up a problem is easy. You just have to be in the right place at the right time and have the necessary know-how. For example I recently witnessed a baby with very low vision have contact lenses inserted into her eyes. There was remarkable change of expression on her face. She abruptly transformed from someone who was not using her vision to someone who was using her vision. She made eye contact with her mother and she immediately started smiling. It was a magical experience. Looking was now a pleasurable activity for her whereas before the contact lens had been inserted the visual sense seemed to lie dormant.

Usually it is a lot more difficult to overcome a problem. This might be because no one really knows what the problem is or, if they do, how to intervene. Each person is individual and unique, so the practitioner needs to try to understand how that particular person is experiencing the world. Seeking to understand the perspective of the participant may provide the key. It comes back to the idea of building on success. A good place to start is to explore how the person is engaging in sense experiences and what types of pleasure he or she is achieving.

There are three distinct types of pleasure. These are: ease, consummatory pleasure and anticipatory pleasure. The key to understanding these three different types of pleasure is an appreciation of the brain's anatomy and evolutionary developmental history.

When you first become acquainted with the anatomy of the human brain it appears enormously intricate and baffling. The evolutionary approach provides one method to reduce the puzzlement. The brain's evolutionary arrangement can be paralleled to the transformation of ancient settlement to modern-day city (Dubuc 2002). Its walled central part established for security in earliest times expands during the medieval ages beyond the city walls to merge with adjacent hamlets. Later a modern conurbation emerges to establish new city limits linked by motorways and the necessary infrastructure required to accommodate the larger more dynamic metropolis of today. In the process modern buildings are built on top of older structures thereby masking earlier settlements.

MacLean's (1990) Triune Brain Theory put forward the idea that the human brain is co-inhabited by three brains: an early reptilian (brainstem, cerebellum and basal ganglia), a later paleomammalian (limbic system) and a modern neo-mammalian (neocortex). Hence the city analogy and like the present-day city, the modern human brain is more intricate than its three parts. A new synergy comes into being.

Scientists estimate it took about 3.3 billion years for the initial single cell organism to evolve into an animal with the first reptilian brain. This originally appeared in fish (about 500 million years ago), then in amphibians (400 million years ago), and finally in reptiles some 320 million years ago, reaching its most advanced stage about 70 million years later. Some claim that the most central parts of the human brain consisting of the brain stem, cerebellum and basal ganglia have similar architecture to the reptilian brain. These parts control essential functions and though reliable, are associated with rigid, compulsive and instinctual behaviours such as dominance, aggression and ritualistic displays.

In his book *The accidental mind* Linden (2007) talks about brain evolution across species and argues that the human brain broadly consists of two parts developmentally: the primitive or 'reptilian' brain, and the more modern brain comprising the limbic system and neocortex. Humans have two sense systems and two emotional systems, one connected to the primitive brain and one connected to the more modern brain. This duality is a particularly important consideration when working with people with brain damage or intellectual impairment.

Ease is associated with the primitive brain. This most basic type of pleasure is a subconscious feeling of comfort and contentment that comes from having essential needs for survival and security met. When people are not receiving sufficient sensory stimulation to generate such pleasure they go into a state of (dis)ease, which is akin to depression. They become agitated. When they are in this state for prolonged periods of time, they may resort to self-stimulation and close off from the outside world of sensory stimulation. The primitive brain, with its own emotional and sensory system, can provide valuable ways to engage with a person, even when there has been debilitating damage to the more modern part of the brain. For example a person with dementia may no longer be able to recognise people, including family members. However they may still be able to enjoy some pleasures such as listening to music.

The second type of pleasure is a conscious experience and is linked to the limbic system. Consummatory pleasure refers to the actual engagement, the consumption or the 'in-the-moment' experience. It is more sophisticated than mere ease because it includes some form of relish of the event.

The third type of pleasure is called anticipatory pleasure and is linked to the neocortex. This comes from looking forward to a repeat of the 'in-the-moment' pleasure experience. This is where we develop an appetite for the sense experience. We desire the sensory gratification. When the practitioner designs an environment where a person can experience an abundance of positive experiences the participant not only enjoys the 'in-the-moment' experience but also looks forward to repeating the experience.

Julie, a teacher of a group of children with profound, multiple disabilities explains how she uses anticipatory pleasure in her teaching.

> My students just love going into the multisensory environment. It's a room we have simply for controlled multisensory stimulation. Going into this room is a high point of their day. Every time we wheel their wheelchairs towards the room they start to vocalise enthusiastically and wave their arms in the air. Often we have to wait outside the door for the room to be cleared and while we're waiting the excitement steadily increases. This seems to make the visit even more enjoyable for them. It's quite contagious. They all excite each other. The longer we have to wait the more excited they become. In some ways it's my favourite part. It's quite an enchanting experience.

Happiness is different to pleasure because it refers to a state of wellbeing, a general feeling of satisfaction. Happiness, however, comes from the person having engaged in pleasurable experiences. The pleasurable experiences make the person happy. It is interesting to observe how happiness is often linked with the idea of flourishing. Happiness therefore is a disposition (a way of being) that supports thriving. Pleasure leads to happiness and happiness leads to flourishing. The condition of happiness provides an ideal situation for the person to grow and develop.

According to Klein (2002, p. xv): 'Our brains have a special circuitry for joy, pleasure and euphoria – we have a happiness system. Just as we come into the world with a capacity for speech, we are also programmed for positive feelings.' What is more, both our thoughts and our emotions alter our brain anatomy and function. Klein (2002, p. xvi) argues that 'with the right exercises we can increase our capacity for happiness' and emphatically concludes 'there is no longer any doubt: we can learn to be happy' (p. xx).

In keeping with this idea that we can learn to be happy Klein (2002, p. xvi) goes on to state that 'our happiness depends at least as much on our environment and our culture as on our genes'. He describes happiness as the brain's signal of a promise of benefit. A person is happy when that person perceives something good is about to happen. It is therefore closely related to the idea of prediction.

Prediction is different to a forecast. A forecast is more general and tends to offer a range of possible outcomes whereas a prediction identifies an expected outcome and so is much more specific. Prediction plays a vitally important role in our daily lives because it enables us to expertly plan what we are going to do. Still it is a difficult skill because there is always going to be some uncertainty regarding future events.

So far in this chapter we have talked about learned optimism and how success breeds success. The more success we experience the more likely we are to make predictions that we will continue to be successful. We also learnt that the opposite, learned helplessness, influences predictions. If we experience a disproportionate amount of failure, and we have no control over that failure, then this will influence our predictions into the future. Furthermore there is a connection with pleasure and happiness.

According to Clark (2008) the idea of prediction also provides us with a key to help us better understand how the brain and the senses work together to make contact with the world. This idea is called Predictive Coding.

Predictive Coding

Predictive Coding, according to Clark (2011), is the proposal that the brain is 'an engine of prediction'. The brain 'exploits prediction and anticipation' to interpret incoming signals and 'to guide perception, thought and action'. As he explains:

> The basic idea is simple. It is that to perceive the world is to successfully predict our own sensory states. The brain uses stored knowledge about the structure of the world and the probabilities of one state or event following another to generate a prediction of what the current state is likely to be.
>
> (Clark 2011)

The concept of Predictive Coding initially appeared in computer science as a method of data analysis based on mathematical principles and models of probability. It has subsequently been adopted by the discipline of computational cognitive neuroscience and used to provide a new model to understand how people use their senses to make contact with the outside world.

Predictive Coding is different to earlier models of perceptual processing. Gibson's (1966) Bottom-Up Theory of perceptual processing was based on the assumption that perception begins with the stimulus and directly flows from the sense organ to the brain, and along the way undergoes successively more complicated forms of analysis. Consequently it was called a direct theory of perception. This is a valid model of how we experience the world but it may not be the major paradigm.

Predictive Coding is the reverse of the Bottom-Up Theory. With Predictive Coding:

> For the most part, we determine the low-level features by applying a cascade of predictions that begin at the very top; with our most general expectations about the nature and state of the world providing constraints on our successively more detailed (fine grain) predictions.
>
> (Clark 2011)

Big picture appreciation precedes any more specific analysis.

Predictive Coding also differs from Gregory's classic Top-Down Theory (Gregory 1970). In this Constructivist Theory, the information that surrounds the stimulation being processed provides extra knowledge as to how the stimulation might be interpreted. Perception therefore involves the combination of information from the sense organ and information stored and processed from past experiences. These then combine to inform the construction of a hypothesis. This theory is now thought to be valid but limited.

Although the Top-Down Theory and Predictive Coding are similarly based on the assumption of the person using contextual information to aid understanding, Predictive Coding is much broader in its conception. The first difference is that Predictive Coding is anticipatory, rather than merely responsive. The second difference is that it extends to the whole body not just the brain. Marstaller (2009) calls Predictive Coding 'an extended mind thesis' because 'the whole body rather than the mere brain should be seen as the locus where sensing and acting come together and allow cognitive systems to engage with the world'. Technological adjuncts, such as virtual reality, further extend the world/cognition interface.

A more complex description of Predictive Coding comes from Clark (2008). He writes that 'certain forms of human cognizing include inextricable tangles of feedback, feed-forward and feed-around loops: loops that promiscuously criss-cross the boundaries of brain, body and world'. This means that '[i]f our minds themselves can include aspects of our social and physical environments, then the kinds of social and physical environments we create can reconfigure our minds and our capacity for thought and reason'. This means our relationship with the environment is even more important than previously acknowledged in earlier theories of perceptual processing. It also helps to explain why Julie's class of children with profound, multiple disabilities got so physically excited about going into their multisensory environment.

Clark (2011) believes that Predictive Coding has four profound implications. The first is that 'good sensory contact . . . becomes a matter of applying the right expectations to the incoming signal'. He maintains because perception is based on the analysis of past perception experiences 'all perception is some form of "expert perception"'. But how does a person develop this expert perception?

Research conducted by Stone and Pascalis (2010) and Stone (2011) gives a clue. They investigated the ability of children to make predictions regarding how visual images were illuminated:

> The shading information in images that depict surfaces of 3-D objects cannot be perceived correctly unless the direction of the illuminating light source is known and, in the absence of this knowledge, perception in adults is consistent with a light-from-above . . . assumption.
>
> (Stone 2011, p. 175)

Results from their research 'suggest that, irrespective of any innate competence, children's ability to interpret shading information is gradually refined throughout childhood' (Stone and Pascalis 2010, p. 1254). This supports the idea of there being a developmental process towards achieving expert perception:

> Children do not see objects in a fully grown-up way until the age of 13. . . . 'Children really do see the world differently to adults, inasmuch as their perceptions seem to be more variable,' says Stone. 'No wonder they can't look at a cloud without seeing a dog or a bear.'
>
> (Fleming 2010, p. 19)

The second implication involves the critical significance of 'the time course of prediction'. Predictive Coding starts with 'the general gist (including the general affective feel)'. If it is accurate then, as time allows, progressively more specific details, both descriptive and affective, are filled in. As Clark observes: 'There is a very real sense in which we properly perceive the forest before the trees' (Clark 2011). Even though Predictive Coding is highly effective at rapidly alerting a person to take evasive action regarding a harmful activity, there is also a down side. If a person has a sensory defensive condition, where a person has a negative reaction to sensory stimulation that is generally regarded as being non-harmful, the initial negative 'general affective feel' may immediately erect an impenetrable barrier, which instantaneously ceases the current engagement.

The third implication is that the boundaries between perception and cognition are distorted. What we perceive is heavily influenced by what we know, and vice versa. This makes us susceptible to 'confirmation bias' (Clark 2011).

This means we are better at identifying evidence that supports our interpretation rather than finding disconfirming evidence. It helps to explain how sensory defensiveness can persist over extended periods of time and the perpetuation of all future non-engagement with similar stimuli.

Clark's fourth implication is the idea that the suppression of prediction errors can lead to the maintenance of the status quo. This is especially evident when a person experiences sensory defensiveness. The affective aspect of the prediction has become so strong that it overrides the sensory processing to such an extent that it prevents the person from engaging in the sensory experience. This has enormous implications for people with learning disabilities, like the residents of the village who lack a positive affect and therefore do not actively seek out engagement with the outside world.

Gaining a better understanding of the four implications of Predictive Coding therefore can provide us with strategies to help people with sensory defensiveness and other sensory and perceptual issues. These will be investigated further in the following chapter.

Chapter 4

Making sense

A developmental process

Introduction

In Chapters 1 and 2 the focus was on the journey multisensory stimulation takes from the sense organs through the nervous system to the brain, and back to the body parts. The term sensory processing was introduced to refer to that fascinating blurred interface where a sense ends and perception begins. Even from these two chapters it is clear that a static assumption of responsiveness to the sensory stimulation is inadequate.

With the introduction of Predictive Coding in Chapter 3, we learnt that the whole process is much more dynamic, with the brain using anticipation to come out to meet the sense stimulation. Rather than the brain solely being the centre of control as was previously assumed, now the entire neural network throughout the body becomes the locus. The concept of Predictive Coding underlines the vital importance of prior experience, particularly success, pleasure and happiness and the reward pathways in the brain. The prediction goes beyond mere description to also include a powerful affective component. If we predict the experience will be unpleasant, then we will be much less likely to want to engage in it, but also vice versa.

Predictive Coding gives a whole new dimension to understanding what constitutes meaningful and rewarding experience. A challenging implication of Predictive Coding is the idea that 'all perception is some form of "expert perception"' (Clark 2011). This indicates there must be some developmental process after birth for the person to achieve this expert status. Becoming an expert does not just happen: it can be disrupted. This chapter concentrates on that developmental process from birth through to just before acquiring perception expert status. It is about how we start to learn to make sense of our world. It is during this developmental process that many children and adults with sense impairments, behavioural problems and learning disabilities first start to demonstrate difficulties.

To help elucidate how sense-learning development takes place I like to use a metaphor of the construction of a bridge across a wide river, which divides two settlements. Each settlement has developed separately. Even though there is some interaction between the two, it is difficult and people tend to stay on their own side. For example a person may row across in a small boat, but only when the weather is favourable.

The bridge is built to a master plan with two spans simultaneously assembled from either bank inwards. When the bridge is finally complete the two spans come together to create a unified whole. This is when the bridge is able to fully function as a conduit between the two settlements and fast-flowing traffic begins to go back and forth across the bridge. Suddenly the two separate settlements operate as a single community. This precipitates an enormous amount of integration between the two settlements and a new level of sharing emerges. The two settlements become one big, highly integrated city.

The same can be said about the developmental process. The developmental process is like building a bridge between the sense organs and the brain and between the brain and the sense organs. On one side there is the bottom-up process. On the other side there is the top-down process.

This two-way bridge enables the brain to work much more effectively and much more efficiently with the body to synthesise sensing, perception, thinking, rewards and acting. Even though there was some communication occurring between the various parts before the bridge was built, it is not until the sense-learning developmental process has taken place that Predictive Coding is able to commence in earnest.

Getting started

Once a baby is born, intense sense-learning development begins with the baby being introduced to novel sensory experiences. At this time there is a tremendous innate propensity for growth, development and learning. At birth a process of synaptic pruning begins where only those neurons that are used survive. This process of synaptic pruning, even though it continues throughout the life of the individual, is particularly active early on in life. The adult brain apparently retains only about 41 per cent of the total number of neurons present at birth (Abitz et al. 2007). This pruning process removes neurons not being used or are damaged, and regenerates and replaces others to achieve much greater synaptic efficiency.

Our genes and the environment both play vital roles in this synaptic pruning process. As Ratey (2001) says: 'everything we do affects the activity of our genes' (p. 32). The environment, or the way we interact with it, 'actually changes the physical interconnection of synapses within the brain' (p. 31), and continues to change this physical interconnection throughout our lives. This interaction between the environment and our genes provides us with the potentiality to not only be responsive but to also make predictions. The foundations for this capacity to make predictions are present from the very beginning. However we need to go through a developmental process of achieving greater synaptic efficiency before it can take full effect.

A novel sensory experience is one that the baby has not yet previously encountered. Indeed for the neonate virtually every experience is new. The baby might react to the novel sensory experience in at least seven possible ways. These reaction possibilities are also relevant for children and adults with sense development issues. Considering them provides us with possible insight into how to design appropriate intervention approaches.

The first reaction possibility is for the baby to simply ignore it. The ignoral is not intentional. It just means the baby shows no signs of awareness of the sense stimulation. It does not register with the baby. Assuming the baby is not fast asleep, the baby is either not paying attention, paying attention to something else, has some kind of sense impairment or learning disability that interferes with sense acuity or sensory processing, and/or the intensity of the stimulation is insufficient to rise above the detection threshold. Whatever the reason, the result is the baby remains oblivious to the sense stimulation, at least at a conscious level. At birth it is natural to ignore the majority of sense stimulation in the environment. It protects the baby from becoming overwhelmed. The neonate spends most of his or her time sleeping.

The second reaction possibility is for the baby to have initial contact and immediately withdraw. This reaction indicates that the stimulation was sufficient in intensity to go over the detection threshold. Withdrawal ensures the baby does not have to endure a repeat performance of the experience, for the time being. This means the novel sense experience, while above the detection threshold will remain under the recognition threshold.

An example of this withdrawal might be an encounter with bright light. The baby sees the bright light but finds the experience unpleasant so the eyes are closed immediately. The baby has not yet learnt to squint when looking at a bright light. The baby does not yet feel sufficiently secure to take a risk with the experience. This very early period of sense development is a particularly vulnerable time because it is when imprinting occurs.

Imprinting is a type of learning that occurs at a phase sensitive time, such as during initial development, which results in a behavioural pattern being established. Here we are not just talking about development by itself. It is the combination of development and learning that establishes a resultant behaviour pattern. Lorenz (1952) used the term imprinting to describe a process observed in goslings hatched in an incubator where they would follow the first moving stimulus they encountered, most notably his boots. The term was introduced into the child development literature in the 1960s to refer to the process by which the baby learns who is his or her mother and father. However it is also applicable to any sensitive moment in child development such as very early sense development when behaviour patterns are being established.

If the baby's environment is harsh – perhaps a result of trauma, illness, neglect, abuse, sense impairment or learning disability – then withdrawal from a sense experience may become a regular reaction to all future novel sense experiences.

This is because the baby has already started to predict that new experiences are going to be overwhelming, unpleasant and/or lack meaning.

Remember Janine in Chapter 1, the eight-month-old infant who was deaf and blind. When I first met her she reacted to each novel sensory stimulation experience by withdrawing. I was foreign and my foreignness stayed that way. No matter what I did, she would withdraw. Furthermore her strenuous protests effectively blocked out any further novel sensory stimulation experience. Janine just tolerated the familiar experiences of being fed and cleaned by her mother, but she vehemently withdrew from any novel experience. It took Janine's parents and myself six weeks of intervention before she started to open up to the possibility of taking in a novel experience. When Janine did stop crying, her reaction was very similar to the third reaction possibility.

The third reaction possibility is for the baby to be curious but wary. Now the baby observes tentatively but from a safe distance, so he or she is not actively involved. This reaction indicates that the baby is feeling somewhat open to a novel experience as long as it is not too close, too intense or overwhelming. Keeping the sensory experience at a distance means that he or she can check it out first before choosing to become more involved.

An especially important characteristic of this type of engagement is that the baby needs to freely choose to engage. Therefore at this very early stage, the novel stimulation must be gentle and unchanging – like an invitation. It needs to pass just over the detection threshold and remain the same. So there must be a very deliberate process of offer and then a deliberate period of waiting for the baby to accept. Any change to the stimulation would make the experience different and that especially includes talking. Change creates a new sense experience and a new sense experience would most likely overwhelm the baby and result in definite withdrawal.

Keeping the stimulation the same without any interference or modulation provides the baby with sufficient time and space to check it out before deciding, freely choosing to become more open to it. The person presenting the novel sense experience needs to respect the baby's need for space and patiently wait for the baby to respond in a positive way. Not waiting for the baby to make the next move could push the baby back into reaction possibility two. This would then make it more difficult next time you try to introduce a novel sense experience.

The fourth reaction possibility is for the baby to find the novel experience pleasant and therefore choose to actively engage with the stimulation. For the baby to be brave enough to take a chance on the new sense experience, the baby must feel comfortable and quietly confident (at ease). This means the baby has had sufficient of their basic survival and security needs attended to. It also means the majority of previous sensory experiences have been positive, so the baby is starting to predict that novel sensory experiences are worth engaging in. They are gratifying.

This is congruent with Erikson's (1950) first stage of psychosocial development. He called this stage 'hope: trust versus mistrust'. During this stage, from birth to twelve months of age, the infant either learns to trust sense experiences or to mistrust them. On the trust side, the infant learns that sense experiences satisfy needs, are dependable, reliable and pleasurable. Alternatively on the mistrust side, the infant learns that senses experiences do not satisfy needs, are not dependable, are not reliable and are unpleasant.

To be successful it is therefore vitally important for the presenter of the novel sensory experience to try to imagine what it is like from the baby's perspective. Try to design a sense experience that is positive, relevant and logical for the baby. By that I mean one that matches the baby's capability and stage of development and interest. For example a simple, natural sense experience for a baby is putting your face close enough to the baby so that it is in the infant's line of vision and then gradually smiling. This begins the visual bonding process. Research tells us that the neonate naturally shows a visual preference for the human face and an auditory preference for the human voice. Once you have the baby's attention you can gradually build on this action, for example by using a higher or lower register to quietly say 'Hello'.

Research tells us that early sensory experiences that the non-disabled baby prefers are taste (particularly the taste of the mother's milk and similar sweet tasting formulas), smell (the mother's milk and associated odours), vestibular stimuli (gentle rocking and movement), and human touch (face on the mother's breast and being wrapped in swaddling clothes to create a feeling of security). We therefore need to design early sense experiences to be congruent with early preferences.

The non-disabled baby at birth can hear, but prefers to listen to the human voice up close. The baby tends to ignore more distant sounds especially ones that are non-human. We also know that initially vision is blurred and only gradually becomes more clear and sharp over time and with usage. There are many visual skills for the baby to learn. For example learning to adjust the eyes to the amount of light, to detect movement, form, shape and perspective. It all takes time and experience. To start off vision is limited to a narrow close range of about 20 cm (both distance from the eyes and area of gaze). That is why the human face is just right as an object of vision for the newborn baby.

It takes up to two months before the infant is able to track a full 180 degrees. Also it is not until four months of age that colour vision starts to develop and even later (about eight to ten months) for depth perception to emerge. It also takes some time for the infant to gain control over his or her head and to achieve hand–eye coordination.

Close observation of the baby will give you valuable information about the size of his or her sense world and enable you to design the most appropriate sense experiences. As the baby grows, develops and learns to use the senses, the size of the baby's sense world also expands. It is important to be aware that for children with sense impairments, learning disabilities and developmental delays, the size of the child's sense world may be much smaller than other children of the same age. That is why it is so important to use observation to work out precisely what is the person's sense world size.

The fifth reaction possibility is an extension of the fourth and is for the baby to become fascinated. Here the baby continues engagement with close attention for an extended period of time. If the baby is fascinated with your smile this is an excellent inroad. The fascination suggests that the sense experience has started to become gratifying in some way and it is the gratification that will motivate the baby to want to continue to engage with the experience. Fascination indicates the sense experience is just right for the baby's stage of development. It is not too easy nor too difficult, not too bright, too loud, too intense – just right.

Typical fascination follows an engagement curve where the attention goes up, plateaus for a while and then subsides. The continued focused engagement is what makes the experience more memorable for the baby and this level of concentration is what is necessary to get the stimulation over the recognition threshold. For babies with a sense disability it may take some time for the attention to go up, to plateau and to subside so in this scenario we need to be particularly observant and patient. If the baby does not engage, then the stimulation is not appropriate.

In Chapter 2 we learnt that smell fades after a person has been exposed to it for a period of time. The phenomenon is called olfactory fatigue. Olfactory fatigue occurs because the person has become accustomed to that particular smell. Each of our senses should undergo fatigue when an unchanging sensory experience is presented. This fatigue helps to explain why our engagement with a particular sensory experience subsides on the engagement curve. Of course once the sensory stimulation has risen over the differential threshold then it is possible to start to change the sensory stimulation in intensity or duration or both, and these changes can reignite the person's attention and extend the plateau.

However if the stimulation does not change in any way and the baby's engagement with that stimulation does not fade then there is a problem of some kind. While a lack of engagement with sensory experiences will lead to sensory deprivation, excessively prolonged engagement with unchanging sensory stimulation will lead to the sixth reaction possibility.

The sixth reaction possibility is for the baby, child or adult to become obsessed with the sensory stimulation. Instead of the sense experience merely providing a gratifying experience, the individual has become fixated on the sensation. The engagement goes up and when it reaches its peak, it stays at that level and does not subside. Because the attention reaches a high and becomes entrapped, the baby is unable to withdraw from the sensation and to move on to another activity.

Donna Williams in her autobiography *Autism and sensing* gives us insight into how this happens. She describes her memories of her early childhood experience of the senses as: 'no interpretation was happening, no judgement, no thought'

(Williams 1998, p. 53). Her experience of the senses was above the detection threshold but below the recognition threshold. She was unable to interpret the sense experience. This lack of interpretation meant her sense experience was just that, a sense experience, nothing else, 'purely a collection of sensations, of sensory impressions' (p. 14). She recalls a particular sense experience with a chandelier where she became fixated on the light:

> I would resonate with the sensory nature of the object with such an absolute purity and loss of self that it was like an overwhelming passion into which you merge and become part of the beauty itself. It was the ultimate in belonging and 'company'. The feeling was completely compelling and addictive.
>
> (Williams 1998, p. 15)

Donna talks about not being aware of a difference between her self and the sense experience. She reasoned that she lost her self because there was no barrier between the two.

It is interesting to reflect on Mahler et al.'s (1975) portrayal of the first few weeks of a baby's life, which they described as a 'normal autistic phase', one where the sense experience and the baby are one. It is like Donna was trapped in this phase. Mahler et al. believed the baby then moves into a 'normal symbiotic phase', which lasts until about five months of age. During this phase the symbiotic relationship narrows to the mother and child. It is this narrowing that helps the sense stimulation be recognised as being separate from the self and mother. From five months of age the infant then moves into a 'separation-individuation phase' where there is a rupturing of the shell between the mother and child. During this phase the infant becomes aware of an outside world. This is a world 'outside-of-self', a sensory world to make sense of. It is a sensory world that can have meaning and significance.

Reflecting her psychological development, Williams (1998) identifies three phases she went through, which she names as 'the sensory . . . the literal . . . and the significant' (pp. 15–17). The sensory is the merging of the self with the sense experience, not knowing there is a difference. This was her 'obsessed with lights' phase. The literal involves recognition of the sense experience for what it is but a lack of depth of awareness of its significance or meaning. A tragicomic example of this is where I once gave a child with learning difficulties a two-dollar coin and told him it was for lunch. Little did I imagine he would take me literally and eat the coin. Other examples of a literal interpretation without under-standing the significance is when a child makes a mud pie and then eats it or a child bites into a 'cake' of soap when having a bath. These actions indicate that the infant does not yet understand the 'significance' of the experience. The third phase is when the infant gains an understanding at a meta-cognitive level, when the child thinks the idea of pretending to eat the lunch money, the mud pie or the cake of soap is hilarious. The child is able to swap over from the literal interpretation side to the significant interpretation side and understand the incongruity being exposed when the swap is made.

The seventh reaction possibility occurs if the stimulation that elicited the obsessive response is continually fed to the individual over an extended period of time. This then results in the person developing an excessive psychological dependence on the stimulation and the person becomes unable to function independently without it. The person becomes addicted to a particular type of sense experience. Of course the more addicted the person becomes to the sense experience, the more the person seeks and requests the sense experience and so a feeder relationship develops between the child and the carer. Sometimes the carer might think the sense experience is appropriate because it helps to make the child more satisfied. The dysfunctional response needs to be recognised.

DeGrandpre (2000) in his book *Ritalin nation* argues that the fast pace of life in the western world, what he calls 'rapid fire culture' has resulted in a pandemic of 'sensory addiction' in children. The particular type of sensory addiction he is talking about is speed of audio-visual stimulation. Through visual technologies such as television, computers and video games, very young children are fed extreme levels of sensory information:

> The 'ADD' [attention deficit disorder] child is of course the perfect example of the need for constant sensory consumption. Studies have documented, for example, how most hyperactive, attention deficit children turn into everyday, normal children under sensory-rich conditions. They have shown how these children begin to fall apart when the sensory stream begins to fade. They have also shown how, under suboptimal sensory conditions children are calmed by the backdrop of stimulation that Ritalin so elegantly provides.
>
> (DeGrandpre 2000, p. 8)

He goes on to controversially argue that Ritalin is merely an addiction substitute, parallel to the use of morphine to combat heroin addiction.

An additional, eighth scenario regarding a possible response to stimulation, which has application not to babies, but to people with sense impairment, autism and learning disabilities, involves stereotypy. Another term for stereotypy is self-stimulation or 'stimming', so named because the behaviour is thought to provide some form of sensory stimulation to the person. There are many different forms of stereotypical behaviours. For example a person with vision impairment might apply pressure to an eyeball while gazing at a light source or rock back and forth incessantly. A person with autism might continually flap both hands. Apart from producing a sensory stimulation experience the repetitive ritual(s) usually appear to be purposeless. Sometimes, however, the behaviour is a way to avoid engaging in other sense experiences, particularly ones that the person is not able to control. Sometimes the behaviour might provide a way of getting ready to do something, and sometimes it just seems to be a behaviour that fills in space when the person is otherwise unoccupied. Stereotypy is discussed in depth in Chapter 8.

As there is very little change in the ritualised behaviour or the sensory stimulation produced, the expectation is that there would be sensory fatigue over time. The fact that this does not occur even though the behaviour may be repeated several thousand times a day suggests that at one level the person may not even be aware they are doing the behaviour. It also suggests that the repetitive behaviour has become their norm, the place from which behaviour starts. Another possibility is that the stimulation does not follow the normal engagement curve. Instead the engagement rises and continues to plateau thereby entrapping the person in the sensation. Stereotypy therefore may be an offshoot of the sixth reaction possibility.

Children and adults with sense impairments, behavioural problems and learning disabilities are clearly more susceptible to developing sensory compulsions, addictions and getting trapped in stereotypical behaviours. As many of these behaviours emerge during the sense-learning developmental period it is particularly important to gain a better understanding as to how this development occurs.

Halliday's triptych

There are useful parallels between the way we learn language and the way we learn to use our senses. One pertinent model comes from a triptych put forward by Halliday (1979). Although it was originally proposed to explain the development of language-learning in young children, it is also relevant to the development of the senses, perception, thought, rewards and action.

A triptych is a work of art that consists of a middle piece, to which left and right panels are attached by hinges. When open, the outside panels are angled to face in towards the viewer to form a complete tripartite work, thereby generating a synergy that would not be possible with just a single part. Triptychs were popular in medieval times. They depicted religious themes and were often made of carved ivory, gold and precious jewels. The three panels meant they could be quickly folded up for safe, easy transportation and even for concealment if necessary.

The three parts of Halliday's (1979) language-learning triptych, are called: 'of', 'through' and 'about'. According to Halliday (1979) language-learning begins with the child acquiring language capability, that is, the learning 'of' the language. For example the child learns that a word has a meaning. This is an operational stage of development. Once the child has learnt the words then the language becomes a vehicle 'through' which further learning can occur, so it reaches the interpretative stage. For example the words can now be used to convey meaning, that is, to communicate with another person. As a consequence learning 'of' and learning 'through' continue to develop simultaneously.

After learning starts to occur 'through' language then it is possible for the child to use that language to reflect on the language being used, and begin to learn 'about' the subtleties of the language. This third stage is a reflective or meta-language stage. For example it is during this stage that the child becomes aware that the meaning of a word may change over time and context. Once the third stage has been introduced all three stages continue to develop simultaneously.

Making sense

The logic Halliday applies to language-learning development similarly applies to sense-learning development. Halliday (1993, p. 93) argues for a 'language-based theory of learning' by saying 'language development is learning how to mean; and because human beings are quintessentially creatures who mean (i.e., who engage in semiotic processes, with natural language as prototypical), all human learning is essentially semiotic in nature'. This includes learning how to use the senses to make sense of the world.

The whole sense-learning development process starts with the learning 'of' the senses. Once again this first stage is operative or pre-interpretative. It is where the child acquires sense-learning capability. This is a time when new pathways are established between the sense organ and the brain. Like learning a language, the learning of the senses is a largely spontaneous and innate process. The baby's brain at birth consists of billions of not yet connected neurons so it is through the child's early experiences that these pathways are established.

A useful analogy might be to think about the way a river forms. The rain falls in the mountains and through gravity the water makes a bed for the water to flow towards the sea. Providing there is enough rain over time the riverbed becomes more pronounced. The learning of the senses is like the riverbed. Once the sense pathway is established then the sense information is ready to flow. However at this initial stage, the learning 'of' the senses, no interpretation is occurring, just the potential flow of information.

If no rain falls in the mountains then no riverbed is formed. Likewise if the baby is blind or is not given access to visual stimuli, then this pathway to the brain will not be established. Also if the baby has very low vision or is only given very limited access to visual stimuli, then the pathway will be tentative. The same kinds of problems may occur with each of the other senses. It is therefore vitally important to prescribe prosthetic devices as early as possible to maximise sense organ acuity. This is because it is the quality and quantity of sense information that helps to establish the pathways to the brain.

The quality and quantity of the sense information is similarly important in the second stage, the learning 'through' the senses. This is the interpretative stage. During this stage there is a three-step process of learning and development that relates to the sense thresholds. When sense stimulation rises above the detection threshold it has the potential to be detected. When sense stimulation rises above the recognition threshold it has the potential to be recognised, and when it rises above the differential threshold it has the potential to become meaningful. This is because the stimulation can be compared and contrasted with earlier bits of information. As we saw before, the thresholds are powerful determinants of a baby's reaction to a novel sensory experience. The build up of prior experience during this 'through' stage is extremely important and memory plays a central role.

Each sense experience begins by laying down the pathway to the brain. We learn to see by seeing. We learn to hear by hearing. The more we use the eyes, or any of our senses for that matter, the better our brain becomes at being able to process that information. When everything is in good working order and the outside world provides a diverse and rich source of stimulation, over time the process of learning 'through' the senses perfects itself, matures. Not only is the person engaging in the sense activity, but now the person has the opportunity to also interpret the sense information.

Learning through the senses means that, in addition to being able to sense, detect, recognise and differentiate the stimulation, some form of meaning is being attributed to the experience. There is synthesis of the information, which includes an affective dimension.

The third stage is learning 'about' the senses, which is a reflective process. This is a meta-sensory or post-interpretative stage. Once a person is able to attribute meaning to a sense experience, the person can start to develop a meta-sensory code or text to better understand what is happening beyond the actual experience. The person can now start to return to their earlier sense experience and re-consider it from different perspectives. This ability to reflect now means the experience can be modified in some way, interpreted and reinterpreted.

For example if you are not able to see a small object you can bring it closer to your eyes to test whether that helps. You might be able to further improve your view by shining a light on the object. Likewise you might be able to improve your ability to smell by putting your nose closer to the source and closing your eyes. Meta-sensory information helps us to start to regulate the way we use our senses. Also it is this ability to reflect on an experience that allows the child to move from what Williams (1998) called 'the literal' to 'the significant' (pp. 32–33).

The bridge is dynamic

Returning to the bridge analogy, the learning 'of' the senses provides the structural materials for the two spans. Brain pathways are being formed. However with the brain, the learning of the senses is a process that never stops. It is like the bridge is always being built with the bridge constantly changing in response to the amount and type of traffic that uses it. Ratey explains (2001, pp. 30–31):

> All of our brains have the same general features that make us human, but each neural connection is unique, reflecting a person's special genetic endowment and life experience. Circuit connections are made stronger or weaker throughout a lifetime according to use. . . . Connections that cope

well with the sensory inputs they receive, which they can convert into effective actions, stay intact and become strong. Those that do not, die off in a process that resembles natural selection.

So the brain bridge is dynamic, with our genes and the environment both playing vital roles in its ongoing construction and maintenance. The learning through the senses opens up the traffic from the sense organs to the brain and in the process starts to build up a pool of experience. The learning about the senses draws on this pool of experience to open up the traffic from the brain back to every sense and motor nerve in the body. When the bridge has traffic moving briskly in two directions anticipation and Predictive Coding become the major determinants of behaviour.

In Chapter 1 we were introduced to the idea of neuroplasticity, which I reported means the brain changes itself in response to the amount and types of stimulation it receives. An important characteristic of neuroplasticity is that it is not always the same. Neuroplasticity during the early synaptic pruning stage is different to neuroplasticity after this has occurred. This is because changes that have happened in the brain in the past influence future changes. The brain changes in many different ways with different processes occurring over a person's life.

With the introduction of Predictive Coding, the description of neuroplasticity needs to be reframed. This is because the brain changes in anticipation of, as well as in response to, the amount and types of stimulation it receives. This anticipation therefore also profoundly influences how the bridge continues to be built and rebuilt into the future.

I described the main principle of neuroplasticity as Hebb's law, which states: 'neurons that fire together wire together' (Doidge 2007, p. 63). This firing can also be anticipatory as well as responsive. Remember in Chapter 3 Julie's class of children were getting excited waiting outside the multisensory environment. This is because they were anticipating that they were going to have an enjoyable sensory experience in the room. The anticipatory pleasure meant that neurons were already firing before the actual experience.

As discussed previously, neuroplasticity challenges the idea that brain functions are fixed in certain locations, opening up exciting possibilities. Reframing in the context of neuroplasticity, Predictive Coding and all their implications highlights the importance of a person regularly experiencing a wide repertoire of pleasurable multisensory experiences. To return to the bridge metaphor there has to be enough traffic on the well-maintained bridge so that the cities on either side function optimally. Once again this has massive implications for people with learning disabilities who only engage with the world when externally motivated and therefore do not achieve their full potential. The challenge is how best to get that traffic flowing.

Chapter 5

Multisensory communication

Introduction

So far we have focused on multisensory processes within an individual, laying the foundation for the rest of the book that will concentrate on the individual's interaction with the wider world. This chapter starts the investigation into that complex process.

To recap, we have learned that during sense-learning development, sense pathways are formed by the flow of sense information from the sense organ to the brain. These pathways continue to be shaped and reshaped throughout the entire life of an individual. If a pathway is not regularly used it soon starts to fade and eventually becomes dormant and vestigial. Conversely with increasing use, the pathway strengthens and becomes more sophisticated.

Through these pathways, a store is built up of sense memories of qualitative and quantitative experiences. This pool of experience promotes further development. Initially the sense experience involves the mere detection of sensory stimulation. With repetition, recognition, differentiation and a meta-sensory understanding become possible. Linkage with reward pathways encourages the individual to make predictions about future sense experiences before they happen.

Chapter 4 is a pivotal chapter because it is during the sense-learning developmental process when many sense-learning difficulties start. These sense-learning difficulties slow down specific and global development, particularly in the area of communication. This is because they inhibit the individual's level and quality of engagement with the outside world. Here we are talking about very early engagement: engagement with sense experiences. These engagements with sense experiences then lead on to engagement with people, objects and events.

We start this chapter with a simple story about a bee and what happens when this bee is inadvertently introduced to a set of novel sense experiences. This story launches our journey into thinking about semiotics, tipping points, issues of multisensory communication and Care Theory.

A bee story

One day a bee flew into my study through a small gap at the top of the window. After flying around the room it tried to leave through the same window except the clear glass window pane barred its retreat. The bee frantically flew up and down the pane searching for an exit. After a while it would fly around the room then it would return to the window and recommence trying to escape through the glass again. Each attempt was just as unsuccessful as the first one had been.

I had been trying to finish something I was working on so at first I was only half aware of the bee. However on its way back to the window it flew quite close to me and I could no longer ignore it. I realised that if it flew into me it would sting me. As I could no longer concentrate on my writing I decided to try to help the bee find its own way out.

I asked myself: 'How can I use what I know about multisensory stimulation to assist?' The bee was currently blocking my access to the window so I closed my eyes and tried to imagine what the space was like for the bee. I quickly realised the room was an internal space – blocked off from the outside and opening into the rest of the house. I could hear the washing machine on its wash cycle and smell food being cooked in the kitchen.

As a result of this observation I closed the study door. This action completely changed the room's ambience. It now felt smaller, more enclosed and quieter. I turned off all the lights. As soon as I could, I opened the window as widely as possible and pulled the curtains back so they did not encroach on the opening. All these actions made a substantial difference to the room's atmosphere. The room felt larger. It connected with the outside world. A gentle breeze wafted in through the window, I could hear street noises and even smell the faint scent of flowers. With the artificial lights turned off the room was now in shade except for a shard of natural sunlight that shone through the open window.

My next move was to position myself in front of the study door with the bee between the window and myself. As the bee continued to fly around the room, by this stage no longer venturing back to the window, my subsequent thought was: 'How can I direct the bee's attention on to the window?' This gave me an idea. I picked up a newspaper and opened it to create a big flat surface. Gradually I vertically raised it to the ceiling thereby substantially reducing the apparent size of the room for the bee. I then slowly moved the newspaper forward and tried to guide the bee in the direction of the window. It worked. All of a sudden the bee changed direction and flew straight out of the window into the garden.

Reflecting on the experience using semiotics

This got me thinking about the bee and its achievement. A bee's brain consists of about 10,000 cells and is the size of a sesame seed. It is minuscule when compared to the human brain. Despite the bee's brain being more than 100 million times smaller, bees share about 30 per cent of their genes with humans, particularly those relating to brain functioning (Weinstock *et al.* 2006). Bees can touch, taste, smell, see and hear.

Furthermore bees communicate with each other and they share important information about their world. Through the so-called 'waggle dance', a successful honeybee forager gives, with the other hive inhabitants, information as to a nectar source, direction, distance from the hive, type and quality (Frisch 1967). Not only do the other bees comprehend the information communicated in the dance, they can remember it in sufficient detail to successfully locate the nectar being described. This means that the dance is essentially tapping into Predictive Coding, aided by being closely associated with a reward.

The bee had been searching for nectar. After the bee flew in through the window it lost its way and in the process it also lost its contact with its anticipated reward. The space inside the study was completely foreign, outside its pool of prior experiences. The bee could not make sufficient sense of the room to work out how to escape. This different set of sensory information translated into the bee experiencing a debilitating sense-learning difficulty. The bee was back to sense detection level, no longer at recognition level. Because the bee was so frantic, it was unable to use the new sense experiences to reorientate and devise new strategies.

The bee had a very limited set of problem solving strategies and when these failed it did not try others. It simply repeated the same strategies over and over again. Furthermore, after a while, even these strategies began to reduce. The bee stopped flying back to the window and it developed learned helplessness.

The closed window did not provide a reward so after several attempts the bee stopped going back to it. This was not habituation; the bee was demonstrating it was capable of associative learning. Associative learning is different to habituation. Habituation occurs when an organism reacts to a stimulus where there is neither a positive nor negative outcome by gradually reducing that behaviour. However in the bee's case the window provided a negative response in so far as it did not enable an escape, so the bee learnt to associate the window with an obstruction.

My job therefore was to try to help the bee overcome its sense-learning difficulty and learned helplessness. I simply provided the right assistance to make it easier for the bee to achieve success. But what kind of assistance did I provide? Was there a particular type of logic to my assistance? I believe there was.

When I decided to help the bee I initially thought the activity was going to be too difficult. After all who tries to communicate with a bee? Most people initially think of communication as being speech and language. Clearly speech and written language were going to be of no use when communicating with the bee. However a broader definition of communication is the conveyance of meaningful information from one being to another, including from human to bee. This broader definition with its focus on the conveyance of meaningful information opened up my options. I could try to communicate using signs.

The scientific study of signs is called semiotics. A sign is any thing – mark, symbol or signal – that stands for something else. In semiotics the focus is on how abstraction is used to communicate. I had already observed that the bee was able to engage in associative learning so I had a possible direction to follow.

I remembered Chaos Theory, which embraces the concept that in dynamic systems simple actions can generate complex unpredictable outcomes (Kellert 1993). I also remembered Complexity Theory where, through dynamics of the tipping point, complex actions can generate simple outcomes (Gladwell 2000). The simple action of the bee flying in through the small space in my study window produced a complex situation for the bee. The bee had entered into a world of novel sensory stimulation and it was overwhelming for the bee.

My goal was to achieve a simple outcome, namely for the bee to escape the room and to independently fly back into the garden, a place it understood. I therefore needed to work out what complex action I could introduce to help make it happen. My objective was to use multisensory stimulation to create a sign that would enable me to communicate with the bee. I wanted to use the multisensory stimulation to deliver a message to the bee, namely how to safely get out of the room. However even that objective was still too hard for the bee to understand. A single sign would not be sufficient. My strategy needed to be even more sophisticated.

Gladwell (2000) talks about how in Complexity Theory a tipping point is located precisely where a significant change takes place. An illustrative example is a bucket on a slight incline perched under a slowly dripping tap. It may take a long time for the bucket to fill and through the pull of gravity to become unbalanced, but eventually there will come an exact moment when just one additional drop is all that is required for the bucket to topple over. This is the tipping point.

This gave me an idea. Instead of providing just one static sign, I could create a series of cascading signs that would help to create an environmental tipping point that would deliver a single message to the bee. The series of signs would funnel the message in ways that would enable the bee to overcome its sense-learning difficulty and independently fly out of the room into the garden. Each of my actions was designed and orchestrated with that final outcome in mind.

I deliberately made changes to the bee's environment so I could deliver the message. I closed the study door, opened the window, drew back the curtains, turned off the lights, stood near the door and used the newspaper to substantially reduce the apparent size of the room. Eventually the bee reached a tipping point and one tiny further change made all the difference. The bee got the message. Immediately the bee flew directly out of the room. The bee had solved the problem and I had been the facilitator. I had managed to use semiotics, multisensory stimulation, Chaos Theory and Complexity Theory to effectively communicate with the bee.

Tipping points

The same method I used with the bee to help it reach its tipping point can also be applied to people with sense-learning disabilities, even though they might have a profound disorder of communication. The key to achieving success is to follow nature's rules. Our sense development is to a large extent hardwired through our DNA. Nature has pre-programmed us with a series of maturational stages, which unfold within a context of nurture, essentially the ambient world. For most of us this is an innate process but for those with sense-learning disabilities actively providing appropriate sense ambiences helps trigger that pre-programmed development potential. So the point here is that we as facilitators are not just trying to communicate any random message. Our communication is very deliberate. It must align with nature's 'roadmap'.

If the practitioner can identify where the person is at (their stage of sense-learning development), what the next stage of sense-learning development is (the goal) then it should be possible for the practitioner to progressively and consistently modify the environment in ways that lead the person towards their tipping point into the next stage. For example a person with brain damage might demonstrate that he or she can detect a particular sense experience but show no evidence of being able to recognise it. This would identify the stage of sense-learning development and the goal to work towards, that is to help the person get over the recognition threshold.

The task therefore would be to design the person's environment in ways that progressively direct the person towards his or her tipping point on the path to achieving recognition. Once the person recognises the sense experience, this recognition provides a basis for communication. Remember it was recognition that enabled me to communicate with the bee. The bee received my message because it recognised a sense experience in the direction of the window. Perhaps it was the faint scent of flowers or the street sounds, but whatever it was the bee recognised it and this recognition was sufficient for it to purposively fly in that direction.

When working in this way it is particularly important that the person with a sense-learning disability freely chooses to engage in the sense experience, that the experience is pleasurable and that there are ample opportunities for repetition, especially once the experience has been recognised. It is best to use a funnel-like approach to deliberately focus the person's attention on the experience and to minimise distractions so the experience itself is unchanging and pure.

It is also important to be mindful that most likely the reason the person has not previously reached this tipping point is because of some previous negative association. Paying particularly close attention to making certain the experience is pleasurable is therefore paramount. Once the person reaches the tipping point then the experience itself takes on a fascination of its own so repeating it will become easier and easier for the person. Moving from one stage to a higher stage is an exciting experience and something the person will naturally want to revisit over and over again so the stimulation has its own motivation. Remember, however, the very first time the person achieves a new skill the locus is still with the old, lower level skill. It is like there is still a gravitational pull back towards the old skill.

Much repetition is needed to help to establish the new skill into the person's behaviour repertoire, for the new skill to develop a momentum of its own. Each repetition helps to solidify the change, for it to become more established. Remember the brain is a use it or lose it organ so repetition and practice are essential. As we have learned before, success spurs on a new wave of development, action and reaction remodelling the person's neural pathways and thereby increasing the sensi-neural traffic across the 'brain bridge'.

Using complexity to generate a paradigm shift in a participant with a sense-learning difficulty offers a lot of potential. It is clearly congruent with the natural way a baby develops. We have already seen that a history of previous success and pleasure helps a baby much more readily reach the tipping point of engagement with a novel sensory experience. Use of tipping points harnesses our innate potential. However if it were just a case of identifying tipping points and activating them through environmental manipulation, our work would be relatively easy.

Chaos Theory applies to biological processes just as much as to mathematics and physics. It helps us to understand how very different outcomes can ensue from seemingly similar simple starting points. Complexity Theory helps us understand how the ensuing chaos can suddenly be resolved into a sharp unified focus. The two theories are a universal duality, constantly tugging at dynamic processes – and this includes responses to multisensory stimulation. Notwithstanding tipping points, the tug of the chaos is ever present.

The goal is success in acquiring a new skill. This opens up a wonderful opportunity for sharing and it provides the motivation to communicate.

Multisensory communication

Multisensory stimulation plays a fundamental role in all communication, as does the need for abstraction, hence semiotics. Communication rests on the need for one thing to signify something else. We learn to communicate through associative learning, being able to associate one thing with another thing. The moment a child's ability level reaches over the recognition threshold, the child has started to make associations, so that this sense experience is similar to the one previously experienced. It is this association that provides the very building blocks of communication. According to Peirce (1931–1958, v. 2, p. 302) 'we think only in signs'. Later he qualified that to include all experience.

Associative learning begins early in humans and links in closely with Predictive Coding. At the olfactory level, for example, we are born smell neutral yet over time our smell experiences and our emotional reactions meld in such a way as to make it virtually impossible to distinguish between the two. A human would find it extremely difficult to objectively smell any odour they found repugnant. The affective component strongly influences the way we perceive the sense experience and prevents us from being able to engage with it in an objective way. However which smells are delightful and which smells are nauseating is highly individual. This very early ability to engage in associative learning is both our strength and our potential downfall. This is because once we begin to associate a sense experience with something negative we are reluctant to engage in it again.

Communication (from the Latin *communicare* 'to share') is defined by *Oxford dictionaries* (2011) as 'the imparting or exchanging of information by speaking, writing, or using some other medium'. Multisensory stimulation is 'some other medium'. However it is not just 'some other medium', it is the first and most basic medium through which information is shared. It is therefore the most important medium we will ever encounter. As a result, a more accurate definition of communication would be the imparting or exchanging of information through multisensory stimulation, speaking, writing or some other medium.

Without multisensory stimulation there would be no communication at all. Multisensory communication is the precursor to speech and language and all higher forms of communication. I think of it as being similar to having one domino knocking another domino over, and so on and so forth in a long string of actions and reactions. When as a result of Predictive Coding, a negative affect towards a sense medium blocks development, it is like a domino that did not fall over. There is blockage. Our job therefore is to try to identify the blockage and provide opportunities for free flow to start to happen. What we need to do is to identify the domino that has not fallen and realign it so it can do its job and knock over the next one.

To learn how to do this we need to have a more accurate understanding of what constitutes communication. Shannon and Weaver (1949) described communication as a simple linear process of information transmission involving five elements, namely: information source (message producer), transmitter (message encoder), channel (medium), receiver (message decoder) and destination. They also added a sixth element at the medium stage called noise (interference).

Despite this model being widely accepted at the time, nowadays it is thought to be overly simplistic. This is because meaning is not merely passively decoded as a simple image of its encoding, possibly debased by some interference. Meaning is constructed. That is why Predictive Coding is so important. The way meaning is constructed is powerfully influenced by context, prior experiences and affective components.

As we have already seen with the bee, multisensory stimulation provides a means by which information is diffused. The scientific study of communication that occurs between non-human species, such as plants, insects and animals, is called biocommunication (Ananthakrishnan and Sen 1998). Biocommunication is predicated on semiotics (Sebeok 1977). With semiotics there is emphasis on signification, regardless of medium or sensory modality (Danesi 1994). Multi-sensory communication therefore fits comfortably in semiotics.

Multisensory stimulation provides the infant with its very first introduction to meaning. Furthermore multisensory stimulation provides the only channel through which communication can develop. Every individual who experiences a difficulty with communication experiences a difficulty with multisensory communication. We learn about meaning by first being able to detect sense information, then recognising it and eventually being able to differentiate it. Right from the beginning, the affective components quickly build to influence the process.

Higher forms of communication such as speech and language require the person to first be able to differentiate sense information. For example with spoken language the person must be able to recognise a sound and then tell whether one sound is different to another sound. Other skills of differentiation involve working out whether a sound is higher or lower in pitch, louder or softer in volume, faster or slower in pace, whether there are longer or shorter pauses between sounds, being able to group sounds together to form words and being able to identify which sounds are given prominence over others. These are all essential skills for the acquisition of spoken language. They take time to develop and they also need to be maintained.

The beauty of multisensory stimulation is that it can be used to communicate even at the most basic levels, for example at the mere detection and recognition levels. Using scaffolding it can help a person develop higher order skills such as differentiating between sense experiences. Successful scaffolding depends on the guiding practitioner being able to determine what ability level the person has achieved and to design intervention strategies that match this ability level. Making the precise match provides the practitioner with a very substantial challenge. To do this the practitioner must be acutely aware of how qualitatively and quantitatively the person is experiencing the world.

We who speak are often so totally addicted to language that we find it almost impossible to imagine what it must be like for a person who does not have speech or language. We use language to think and the way we think shapes our language. Language dominates us and speakers find it almost impossible to divorce themselves from it. That is why semiotics is valuable. This is because semiotics transfers the focus from linguistics onto the meaning of the sign.

In the same way I tried to imagine what it was like for the bee, we also need to try to imagine what the experience is like for a child with sense-learning difficulties. If the child does not speak then we must try to think and communicate in non-spoken ways. If the child is blind then we must try to think and communicate in non-visual ways. If the child is deaf then we must try to think and communicate in non-auditory ways and so on and so forth. This peeling off of higher forms of cognitive processing, ways of thinking, ways of communicating and ways of experiencing the world, helps the practitioner design more precise matches. To successfully communicate with the child we must use information that the child understands. This information comes from the child's own experiences and abilities. These provide the basic vocabulary for communication and our communication must involve making associations between these experiences. There is no other way.

According to the Canadian communication theorist Marshall McLuhan (1964) too much attention is placed on the more obvious content of the communication and not enough consideration is given to the less obvious medium of the communication. He summed up this idea in his famous saying: 'The medium is the message.' McLuhan argues that the message and the medium combine to create an interdependent association with each other so that over time the medium influences the way the message is understood. McLuhan illustrated this using an example of the way distressing news items about violence on television can start to desensitise a person or conversely encourage them to believe their local area is more dangerous than it actually is. So it is not only the content that is important. The medium is also influential. This means that not only does the construction of the message change over time but the medium itself also shapes the way the message is constructed.

A multisensory illustration is the tactile sense and tactile defensiveness. Focusing on the medium, the tactile sense, rather than the message, what is being touched at a particular point in time, may provide us with new ways to address the sense-learning difficulty. One starts to think more about the meta-sensory aspects such as when does the person use touch, how do they use touch, for what purposes, and how do they feel about these touch experiences? Answers to these questions may provide valuable clues to intervention.

There is also an ethical component to multisensory communication and the use of semiotics with a person with a sense-learning difficulty and the fundamental requisite is to help that person find meaning. Multisensory communication needs to be nuanced and it needs to be predicated on an ethical platform. How to nuance is the subject of Part II of this book. Care Theory provides the ethical foundation for multisensory communication and semiotics to proceed. In Care Theory the medium is indeed the message. A key part of this message is that social interaction, particularly in the developmental period, particularly through a caring facilitator, is essential for neuroplasticity to occur (Lin Lu *et al.* 2003).

Care Theory

Care Theory first appeared in 1984 in a book written by Nel Noddings called *Caring: a feminine approach to ethics and moral education*. In it she talks about the ethics of care, that is what makes actions right or wrong. When thinking about multisensory communication it is imperative to consider one's actions to ensure they are ethically defensible. This is particularly germane when using multisensory communication with people with communication disorders who have extremely limited ways of communicating.

Much of what has already been written in this book is about sense relationships. We have examined how the relationship between the affective and the sense experience provides the basis for associative learning and communication to develop. We have also learnt that negative affects associated with particular sense experiences can erect impenetrable barriers that disrupt development. Noddings similarly stresses the indispensable importance of relationships, except she comes at relationships from a different direction. She emphasises the development of a caring relationship as an essential part of caring. For caring to take place she argues there must be the carer, the cared-for and a caring relationship between the two. The exciting point about Noddings' Care Theory is that this caring relationship provides a rescue remedy for those who are experiencing particular sense-learning experiences.

What makes the relationship a caring relationship is recognition on the part of the cared-for that an act of caring has taken place. It is this recognition that makes the difference because the cared-for begins to trust the carer and the cared-for becomes willing to follow the carer in new directions. For it to be caring there must be a degree of reciprocity, that is to say both carer and cared-for gain from the encounter in different ways and both give. My encounter with the bee would not be considered a caring relationship because the bee did not recognise that a caring action had taken place. My communication with the bee consisted of a single message and a single response with very little reciprocity. However it was in the right direction because the relationship resulted in a positive and liberating experience for the bee.

Noddings believes the carer achieves this special relationship with the cared-for through an ongoing process of receptive attention that she calls 'engrossment', a state of continuing complete absorption in the cared-for. With engrossment the carer is as open as possible to what the cared-for is trying to communicate. Here we need to completely turn the table around and use semiotics to try to decipher what the cared-for is trying to signal to us. The carer must constantly check and recheck that the message being received is accurate and that the interpretation remains accurate throughout the interaction. I have already alluded to ways to help with engrossment such as trying to imagine what the experience is like for the person and also trying to respond using signs the person will understand, signs from the person's own vocabulary.

For example a mother of a newborn baby might spend long periods of time lovingly attending to the baby's basic needs in concrete ways and in the process create communication-response opportunities that build on what the baby does. If the mother smiles and the baby smiles back in response, a behavioural-feedback loop is established. The baby is demonstrating awareness that he or she is cared-for. Next time the baby might smile first and wait for the mother to smile. The mother–baby interaction can be interpreted as a form of rudimentary conversation, one where the message is one of caring.

This cared-for state, according to Noddings, provides the optimum environment for learning and development and for remediation if there are problems. Furthermore, as McLuhan would say, the medium itself takes on a quality of caring and becomes the message. Caring then provides the ideal scaffold for sense-learning recuperation and development to occur. Engrossment becomes much more challenging when the cared-for experiences extreme difficulty with communication and has disabilities or conditions that greatly influence the cared-for's state of being.

Like the mother of the newborn child, the carer of a person with a disability begins the process by ensuring that the cared-for's basic needs are being attended to and then gradually refines the communication over time. For Noddings, engrossment begins with the carer's motive energy flowing towards the cared-for. By that she means the carer tries to pick up information about the cared-for's communication motive. The carer works at identifying what the cared-for's purpose or motivation behind the attempt at communication might be. This involves careful contextual observation of behaviour.

A mother tries to guess the newborn infant's communication purpose by logically checking through the baby's basic needs such as comfort, nutrition and sleep. At first it might be a gradual process of elimination but over time both the carer and the cared-for become better and better at refining the communication. The more accurate the carer is at interpreting the message the better equipped the carer becomes at being able to respond in ways that are relevant, helpful and hopeful. Furthermore once the cared-for recognises that an act of caring has occurred, the cared-for becomes more motivated to respond, to continue the communication. This in turn strengthens the feedback loop.

In addition to working through a list of basic needs and initially responding in concrete ways, it is important for the carer to examine his or her own biases and assumptions and put them to one side. For example, people who can see naturally assume that the cared-for can also see. However if the cared-for is blind the carer's response must be non-visual otherwise the response will not be meaningful for the cared-for. If the cared-for has low vision then the response will need to be both visual and non-visual. Similarly if the cared-for is deaf the response must be presented in non-auditory ways, and so on depending on the particular characteristics of the cared-for.

The carer therefore must endeavour to understand the multiple perspectives of the cared-for and respond in ways that take these perspectives into account. Remember if the cared-for does not recognise the carer's actions as caring then they are not caring. The carer must become adept at being able to use a sense-logic as it applies to the cared-for. When Noddings asks: 'What are we like [when we engage in caring encounters]?', we discover that we are receptive and attentive in this highly specialised way. The carer builds up knowledge of the cared-for's skills and abilities through ongoing engrossment, checking and rechecking. Constantly imagining what it is like to be the cared-for, and trying to understand as accurately as possible what the cared-for is experiencing help to kick-start the process.

Noddings believes there are four key components of caring interactions. These are: modelling, dialogue, practice and confirmation. These components take place within the medium of a caring relationship.

Modelling refers to the way we represent something in our own behaviour. Noddings (1995) argues: 'We have to show in our behavior what it means to care . . .We demonstrate our caring in our relations with them.' Parents of very young children manage this by initially copying the child's behaviours.They do this until they have collected sufficient information about what the child is experiencing to be able to build a meaningful response that is within the child's repertoire, something the child will recognise. Of course it becomes much more challenging if the person has a disability.To avert misunderstanding, we need to be highly alert to how the replicated experience appears to the cared-for. So the important point here is that the modelling is one of caring and it is the modelling that becomes part of the caring medium.

By copying the behaviour of the child and reflecting it back to the child the child gains two different perspectives, that of their own action and that of the carer modelling it back to them. This modelling provides the basis of communication because it may be the first time an infant has had their own behaviour reflected back to them. For example observe an infant who is crying and then copy the cry as accurately as possible. Most often the baby will stop crying and observe closely. Once you have the child's attention then it is time to begin the second component – dialogue.

For Noddings (1992) dialogue is part of the lived experience of caring, where we exercise our engrossment. Through dialogue we model caring communication. She says: 'Dialogue is such an essential part of caring that we could not model caring without engaging in it.' As we try to care, the feedback the cared-for gives helps us improve the way we demonstrate it. If we are able to provide the child with a meaningful response and the child responds in kind then this enables the dialogue to continue.

For it to be regarded as dialogue it does not have to involve spoken communication. Dialogue can consist of a series of simple responses. For children with communication disorders the carer must be especially receptive to what the cared-for is trying to communicate for the dialogue to be able to continue in a meaningful way. Remember dialogue is simply the exchange of information. It should be thought of as being multisensorily based, not language based. A description of a simple dialogue is a baby cries, the carer responds by modelling the crying in a caring way, the cared-for responds by stopping crying and observing the carer, the carer responds by stopping crying and modelling the baby's new expression of paying close attention. The cared-for responds by continuing to pay close attention, the carer responds by smiling gently and then the cared-for responds by also smiling gently. The carer then responds by drawing attention to the smile in a confirming way.

If dialogue is bidirectional, the cared-for gets to practise what the carer is modelling. Practice is where the cared-for gains mastery over his or her behavioural repertoire. According to Noddings all children 'should be involved in caring apprenticeships' (Noddings 1984, p. 187). The goal of this communication is to reveal to the student something to nurture, an ethical ideal. For example in the previous example of a simple dialogue the infant goes on a journey from being upset and crying to being able to produce a gentle smile. This journey models to the child how to make a transition from being upset and alone to being with someone else and smiling together.

'When we attribute the best possible motive consonant with reality to the cared-for, we confirm' (Noddings 1984, p. 193). When we confirm something we are identifying a better self and encouraging this better self. When the carer ended the dialogue by drawing attention to the smile in a confirming way, the confirmation is like a form of punctuation. It reaffirms the message, drives it home.

Chapter 6

Design for multisensory stimulation

Introduction

The first five chapters of this book were devoted to thinking about the nature of sense-learning development difficulties and proposing a coherent theory to explain how they occur. Such information is vital to help inform what intervention strategies to use with children and adults who experience difficulties in the sense area. These difficulties may occur because the child has not yet achieved a particular developmental stage or because the person is in regression. The latter is when a person's development stops and begins a reverse cycle, often because of brain damage. When regression occurs the developmental stages continue to provide useful information regarding suitable intervention.

Neural pathways become dysfunctional or even non-functional either through congenital causes or though acquired causes such as neglect, trauma, disease and/or ageing. If rehabilitation does not occur spontaneously through unstructured day-to-day interactions, then structured intervention is required. This structured intervention must be designed carefully to nurture the potential of the individual with the sense disability (Gibson 1977).

Such rehabilitation is often not easy. For the pathways to start working again, the person must willingly engage in sufficient and appropriate sensory stimulation to kick-start the whole process into motion. Convincing the person to willingly engage, especially someone who has lost interest in external stimulation, is a challenge. This is particularly the case when there are problems such as down time (see Chapter 3, p. 24) and ritualised self-stimulation (see Chapter 4, p. 42).

To be able to lead the participant into actively engaging with the outside world the practitioner must have a place where multisensory stimulation can be controlled and managed in ways that continue to appeal to that participant. The remainder of this book concentrates on how the practitioner can use multisensory stimulation with children and adults with sense-learning difficulties. We start this journey into the practical in this chapter by thinking about environmental design, how to create more suitable spaces for sensory engagement.

The rationale

For the individual without a sense disability, the role of the environment and of the carer can almost be taken for granted, or at least that is the way it initially appears. The natural un-engineered environment is abundantly rich with sensory possibility and challenge and this stimulates the seemingly spontaneous sense-learning development described in the first five chapters.

In Chapter 1 we were introduced to the idea of neuroplasticity, the idea that the brain changes in response to the amount and type of stimulation it receives. In subsequent chapters we have learnt five important characteristics of neuro-plasticity. These are:

1   Neuroplasticity is dependent upon use. Sensory stimulation is essential for neuroplasticity to occur. The more multisensory and the more gratifying the stimulation is, the more powerful it becomes.
2   Social interaction, particularly in the developmental period, is essential for neuroplasticity to occur.
3   Neuroplasticity is age related. Different types of neuroplasticity come into play throughout the life span of the individual. From birth a process of synaptic pruning occurs where only those synapses that are used, and continue to be used, survive. After childhood, lack of use of established pathways results in them fading, becoming dormant and vestigial.
4   The nature of neuroplasticity itself changes over time. Changes that have happened in the brain in the past influence the nature of future changes.
5   Two key strands of neuroplasticity are developmental neuroplasticity, which occurs in response to stimulation, learning and memory, and compensatory neuroplasticity, which occurs when one function is lost and another function is introduced to take its place.

When we are thinking about the design of environments for the use of multi-sensory stimulation all five characteristics of neuroplasticity are considered in conjunction with the role of the caring facilitator. As Noddings (1984) reminds us with Care Theory all babies heavily depend upon the quality and type of caring that is provided. This quality of care plays a powerful determining role in early sense-learning development especially through crucial transition stages. So even when the child does not experience any problems with sense-learning development the role of the carer is vital.

In Chapter 4 I used Halliday's triptych to argue that the way the child acquires sense abilities is consistent with the way a child acquires language. Through the process of learning of, through and about the senses the child establishes a pool of experience, which accumulates over time. Recent research suggests that the child becomes sensitive to the distributional frequencies of particular types of sensory experiences being encountered. It is this accumulation of experience that facilitates sensory processing transitions from detection to recognition, and from recognition to being able to make differentiations. Once differentiations are possible then there is an ongoing process of refinement through a steady stream of basic concepts, such as louder, softer, higher, lower, wet, dry and so on and so forth.

According to Kuhl (2007, p. 112), a world authority on early language acquisition, 'infants learn "statistically" – they are sensitive to the distributional frequencies of the sounds they hear . . . and this alters perception'. The important point is this ability to learn statistically is not only dependent upon the accumulation of experience gained by interacting with the environment, but it is also dependent upon social interaction. Transition through 'the earliest phases of language acquisition . . . requires social interaction' (p. 110).

Kuhl and her team exposed a control group of six- to eight-month-old infants to particular language-associated sensory stimuli using television or audio only channels. The infants 'showed no evidence of learning' (p. 114) whereas when the identical information was provided by a physical person to a second group of infants of the same age, learning did occur. This research strongly supports the hypothesis that there are two essential ingredients to early sense development: a suitable environment coupled with a caring facilitator.

It is the combination of the caring facilitator plus the controlled environment that strongly enables the person to make a transition from one stage to another. However there is a third consideration, that of timing. There seems to be an optimal time for these early transitions to occur. This is because of the synaptic pruning that takes place during early development. For example in Kuhl's research the optimal time for infants to be able to distinguish between l and r (in English and in Japanese language acquisition) was between six to eight months. After this age the ability to learn to make such distinctions declines. This means that a person may still learn the skill but it takes much more deliberate intervention. The development can no longer be taken for granted.

The importance of requiring the combination of a caring facilitator and a controlled environment designed to match the participant's interests and needs is particularly relevant for three different groups. They are: children and adults with severe multiple disabilities, children and adults with autism or any other condition where there is an impairment of social interaction, and children and adults with severe sensory setbacks due to disease, neglect or trauma.

Children with severe multiple disabilities experience developmental delay so their stage of development will be considerably slower than their chronological age. However because the synaptic pruning still occurs regardless of developmental stage reached, it will be more difficult for critical transitions in sense-learning development to occur. This is the rationale for specialist intervention. The input of the caring facilitator will need to be much more specialised, much more targeted, much more focused on helping the child achieve these transitions.

Children and adults with autism or other conditions where there is a severe impairment of social interaction will also require more explicit carer input. This is because social interaction is necessary to help the person make a transition from one stage to another. The caring facilitator does this by communicating with the person with autism through the controlled environment. The controlled environment becomes a way to communicate with the individual.

Children and adults who have experienced severe sensory setbacks due to trauma, disease, neglect or abuse also benefit from the input of a caring facilitator. Here the caring facilitator modulates the controlled multisensory environment in ways that are meaningful to the participant. This form of interaction is aimed at promoting brain repair. This means that the person may have previously been able to function at a higher stage but due to regression this skill was lost. More complex challenges for the designer occur when there are different permutations and combinations of factors that impede sense-learning development. These then need to be considered more individually, especially in the context of compensatory neuroplasticity.

For these groups of individuals the natural environment is not enough to trigger learning and development. The individual will make more progress in a controlled environment specially tailored for his or her individual needs by a caring practitioner. The caring practitioner is able to design a less overwhelming environment so it can be pleasurable and, as we have established in Chapter 3, a positive affect is a powerful determinant of sense learning.

Design approaches

The design of a dedicated space for multisensory stimulation is predicated on goals for the space, the likely users, the practitioner mix working in the space, location issues, the socio-cultural context, cost, engineering considerations, aesthetics and even trend spotting. Good design requires considerable research, collaboration and teamwork, attention to detail, drafting and redrafting, creation of models, ongoing adjustment and re-design. It is an active process that continues throughout the life of the dedicated space.

We will now look at six design approaches. They are: user-centred design, function-centred design, simplicity whenever possible, multiple methods to achieve the same outcome, slow design and design prototypes. Each approach provides pertinent information for the designer(s) to consider, both in regard to the physical nature of the space and also how it is used.

User-centred design

'User-centred design' begins by the practitioners identifying who are the users, what are their needs and interests, and becoming aware of their relevant prior experiences. A good way to achieve this is through multi-disciplinary collaboration with all stakeholders in the project. This includes with the participants themselves, whenever possible. The design objective is to ethically tap into participant desires: what gives them pleasure, what makes them happy, what enables them to make sense of their experiences. For example, the user's age will influence the size of the space with a smaller space more likely to suit young children and a larger space more suitable for adolescents and adults, although a smaller space may also be suitable for people with dementia. Users who are not able to independently move around require additional design features such as hoists and ceiling tracks to easily transport them from wheelchair to activities within the space such as a waterbed or ball pool.

Nowadays designers are strongly advised to devise installations that can be used by all people regardless of their ability. This ensures that the space is more flexible should the participant base change over time. It also helps the designer anticipate and accommodate new legislation and policy requirements that will undoubtedly surface in the future as a condition of continued government funding or for registration, accreditation or endorsement.

Function-centred design

In 'function-centred design' the focus of the planning process is to clearly identify all the purposes the space will be required to facilitate. This involves asking all staff planning to use the space to complete an audit of the types of goals and tasks they wish to accomplish. These may include providing facilities to enable the participant to engage in stimulation for leisure and recreation, for therapy and/or for educational activities. Each application opens up a range of specific goals and tasks. These specific goals and tasks, once they have been identified, are subsequently employed to inform the overall design process. Obviously the qualifications, background and discipline interests of different practitioners will influence the types of functions they are likely to identify, so it is vitally important to include them all in the initial design process.

If this level of cooperation does not occur and one person exclusively takes on the design supervisor role without extensively consulting with colleagues, there is real danger the project will fall flat due to the lack of staff buy-in. Conversely, however, when different staff become involved in the design process often the outcome is much richer than it would have been if only one person had been involved. The process of designing the space provides the key stakeholders with an important education, which enables stakeholders to better use the space in the future.

Simplicity whenever possible

When designing a space for multisensory stimulation it is critical to streamline. Identify and eliminate potential unnecessary complications and ensure all the practitioners are easily able to manage the space and operate all equipment. One problem with employing an outside expert to design and construct the environment is that the result may be a lot of complicated features that staff do not know how to use or how to fix if a problem occurs. If that happens, it is inevitable that staff will quickly lose interest and cease to use the space. It becomes a white elephant, an expensive installation, which cannot be easily disposed of yet has little practical usefulness.

Even if an expert is employed, practitioners are strongly advised to make sure they are in full control of the process. Otherwise the outside expert's design might be more dutifully subservient to commercial and technological interests than specifically aimed at catering for the needs of the actual users. So the idea of 'simplicity whenever possible' is to guarantee all practitioner users understand how the space will work and be maintained, while at the same time taking into account all essential aspects such as: workplace health and safety, cleaning, electrical, lighting, sound proofing, storage, accessibility, ventilation, heating and cooling.

The most significant reason for following the simplicity whenever possible design approach though is to ensure that the practitioner is able to work with the environment to help the participant. Remember social interaction, particularly in the developmental period, is essential for neuroplasticity to occur. It is the caring facilitator who uses the multisensory stimulation to help the participant develop and learn. This social interaction continues to play an important role throughout the life of the individual.

Multiple methods to achieve the same outcome

Remember the bee story in Chapter 5, how I used Chaos Theory and Complexity Theory to set up a cascade of environmental changes that enabled the bee to find its own way out of the room? To begin with the facilitator is important. The facilitator plays a key role. If I had not made these changes then the bee would not have located the exit.

The bee story provides a useful illustration of the 'multiple methods to achieve the same outcome' design approach. The approach grew out of my experience of working with people with exceptional needs, particularly those with communication disorders. I discovered that if one strategy set does not appeal to a participant, then another might.

When working with people with multiple disabilities and communication disorders there is an ongoing process of close observation and experimentation, which makes it possible for the practitioner to more precisely zero in on the participant's needs and interests and to identify the next transition to be accomplished. However for this to happen the practitioner requires a particular type of space to support this line of enquiry, one that is different to a simple personal fixed design.

The traditional simple personal fixed design refers to the tendency to plan an unchanging space that compliments the designer's own preferences, ways of experiencing the world, and ways of thinking and understanding. The finished product therefore is a reflection of the designer's personality, interests and capabilities, which might suit the designer but it is less likely to please others.

A better design is one that takes on a floating, more flexible quality and incorporates multiple sense logics to make it possible for the practitioner to design and re-design the space from the participant out, ideally during the actual session. Therefore whatever disability the participant has, the space can be re-configured to accommodate appropriate sense logics.

The idea of a floating design is similar to a floating currency exchange rate. Here the design process never ends. It is always being negotiated and renegotiated. Creating a floating design is a multifaceted challenge because those in the participant population are not only markedly different from those in the general population but they are also markedly different from each other. They are exceptional: they have dissimilar characteristics, abilities and needs. This exceptionality accentuates the need for design flexibility.

To achieve flexibility each design feature is conceptualised along a design continuum. This makes it easy for the practitioner to re-design the space as the need arises. For example, from a visual perspective white is a design neutral colour because lighting can be used to change it to another colour. A second example from an auditory perspective involves the use of soundproofing. This gives the room greater auditory flexibility (see Design prototypes later in this chapter).

The floating design environment is multifunctional. Rogers (1997, p. 10) used Walzer's classification of an 'open-minded' space to describe an area that is flexible enough to be able to cater to a range of different functions or applications. Rogers argues that when a space has a multifunctional capacity the space is more sustainable. The space can transform to cater for a wider range of 'participants' so it is more suitable for sharing and social interaction. Design flexibility makes the environment an active contributor in the sense-learning development process. Mertens (2008, p. 13) describes this phenomenon as a 'didactic triangle' where the participant, the practitioner and the 'designed *environment*' are all active players.

The flexible environment gives the practitioner greater control over constancy and change. This ability to actively manipulate constancy and change becomes a tool to promote participant self-sufficiency and generalisation. When the participant independently works out how to do an activity, then he or she is more likely to replicate it and practise it. When participants work out their own method of doing an activity, then it is more personally meaningful, memorable and open to adaptation once the environment changes.

A key point of the approach is, unlike the regular environment, the design does not corral the participant into a repetitive way of performing an activity. The space is more malleable and acquiescent, less dominant, thereby offering the participant room to negotiate, to play, to make it their own, an experience that might be quite rare in the outside world. Two words to sum up the multiple methods to achieve the same outcome design approach are 'design plasticity'. This design plasticity makes the environment a tool for the practitioner to use to stimulate neuroplastic development in the participant.

Slow design

'Slow design' concentrates on wellbeing: of the individual within the socio-cultural and the environmental context (Fuad-Luke 2004). Just as the Italian slow food movement is a revolt against fast food, so slow design is a revolt against fast design. Fast design (such as seen on reality television makeover shows) is superficial and glib; it focuses on instantaneous materialist outcomes and product placement/free market manipulation of perceived wants. This is particularly pertinent because the design of environments for people with sense-learning difficulties has tended to be dominated by commercial interests with ready-made products, which can threaten the importance of the caring facilitator.

Slow design therefore provides a refreshing alternative. Slow design with its focus on wellbeing has the long-term goal of catering to the real needs of real people. Furthermore, because one of the goals of slow design is to incorporate as many relevant features or 'flavours' as possible, all four previously mentioned design foci, namely: user, function, simplicity and multiple methods to achieve an outcome, can readily be included.

Slow design enthusiasts look to positive psychology theorists to inform their planning decisions. These include Seligman (1975, 1998) who writes on learned optimism (see Chapter 3, p. 27) and Csikszentmihalyi (1998). Csikszentmihalyi asserts that people are most happy when they are in an environment that enables them to become absorbed in an activity that makes a match between task complexity and sense capability. This also fits nicely with the idea of a floating design.

Because the central focus of slow design is on human wellbeing, the issue of human needs is paramount. These include physical, emotional and social needs as well as mental health considerations. Slow design enthusiasts often start with Maslow's (1954) hierarchy of needs. These are presented in the shape of a pyramid with the base consisting of the most basic requisite physiological needs such as breathing, food, water, sleep and homeostasis. These must be attended to before the person is able to move up the pyramid to higher needs such as safety, love/belonging, esteem and eventually self-actualisation.

Design prototypes

Having decided to create a dedicated space for multisensory stimulation, practitioners often have considerable uncertainty as to what types of areas would best suit their current and future participants. They begin to toy with possible designs that are within their own experience, spaces they have actually worked in or visited. While not without value, this approach is limited in scope because it is often strongly dominated by the visual sense.

To help illustrate just how strong visual dominance can be I want to share a story about when I was a consultant for a craft group that was producing tactile illustrations for children who were blind. One task involved making a tactile glove for the cover of a tactile book. The outside of the glove was to be in cotton and inside the glove there would be a distinctly different tactile surprise for each fingertip to discover. I introduced the concept and asked the particular craft person to experiment to try to find out which texture would best suit each finger, for example kid leather feels wonderful if explored by the little finger. I then left her to prepare the glove using her own design. The final product shocked me. She decided not to make a glove. Instead she made a visual imprint of a hand on a black background with each finger represented by a different coloured piece of the same textured cotton material. They all felt exactly the same. Even though it was interesting visually it did not follow a tactile logic at all. I said: 'This is supposed to be for children who cannot see. Each finger feels the same.' The volunteer told me: 'I know but I'm a visual person and I just could not make an item that was not visual. It's the cover of the book. I had to make it visual.'

This same problem occurs when trying to design environments for the use of multisensory stimulation. According to Blesser and Salter (2007) there is an absence of understanding of different forms of sensory architecture. This is because, in addition to architects designing in visual ways, much of the terminology to describe space is visual. Visual concepts therefore keep on hijacking the design concept. Classen (2005) calls it a visual paradigm. The way we sense is the way we understand so if vision is our dominant sense then we have a world 'view'.

Classen (2005, p. 160) believes there are many different 'sensory paradigms'. A paradigm is a framework within which operates a certain set of thinking and practices. One dictionary definition I found described a paradigm as a 'world-view', an unfortunate definition, which only reinforces my argument that visual language dominates the way we think. The prototype is an attempt to create a space that follows a particular sense paradigm. It is important to remember that these sensory paradigms are incommensurable, which basically means they cannot be reconciled (Kuhn 1996). It is like comparing apples with oranges. To be able to design non-visual spaces we must be able to think about space in non-visual ways and develop non-visual terminology to describe this space.

My introduction to aural architecture occurred during a visit to Australia's capital city Canberra with a friend who is congenitally blind. We agreed I would guide her through the National Art Gallery and she would guide me through the High Court, a building she knew and loved. As we approached the High Court I closed my eyes, held her elbow and she led me up the long, paved ramp, past the soothing white noise trickles of the waterfall, and into the imposing Public Hall. As soon as we entered it I could tell it was a magnificent space, just by the resonance of the sounds it produced. I could hear sounds reflecting off the 24-metre high ceiling, the solid concrete walls, the glass front, the extensive wooden panelling and the marble floor. I was astonished at how clearly I could hear the space. Each element came together to create a wonderful aural experience that exuded such strength and security.

I realised that if I had kept my eyes open I would have completely missed the aural experience because it would have been subjugated by the visual. My friend had introduced me to a new way of experiencing the building. Even though I have spent many years teaching children who are blind sometimes the only way I can think in non-visual ways is to close my eyes and to keep them closed. Otherwise the visual takes over and I forget to consider a location from other sense perspectives. So the idea of the design prototype is to create an environment that provides an 'affordance'. An affordance is a term proposed by Gibson (1977) to refer to the quality of an environment or set of circumstances that allows a person to perform an action, so it is an action possibility.

I developed a set of design prototypes (Pagliano 2001) to help overcome the problem of visual domination when designing sensory environments. A prototype is an original model. Each prototype is a model of a particular design concept for the dedicated space. The design concepts aim to deliver different strands of multisensory stimulation in a pure form. The value of a prototype is that it elucidates the basic ideas behind each specific design. The designer is then able to combine different design prototypes into the one space, thereby producing a hybrid environment, one that incorporates a number of different types of experiences to cater for an even more diverse group of participant needs.

Each basic design prototype has its own design features and a rationale that links back to research and theory in ways to help the practitioner make informed but practical decisions when choosing a final design. The seventeen basic design prototypes are: olfactory space, interoception space, white room, dark room, grey room, acoustically sharp sound space, acoustically dull sound space, tactile space, gustatory space, interactive area, water area, soft play, portable environment, virtual environment, inclusive area, pluralist environment and social space. Finally I need to emphasise the point that each prototype is merely a tool of the practitioner, a way to communicate with the person with a sense difficulty. Without the practitioner, the space is of little value.

Olfactory space

The olfactory space specialises in providing stimulation for the sense of smell. This is the most complicated prototype to design. Smell has convoluted psychological overtones that make it extraordinarily powerful and pervasive. This is because we are born smell neutral and our early affective experiences shape how we interpret particular smells. Pleasant experiences link with smells we regard as pleasant and unpleasant experiences link with smells we regard as unpleasant. Over time they can become exaggerated and out of balance so one goal of the olfactory space might be to help the person rebalance their engagement with smell.

When designing an olfactory space we need to constantly remember that some individuals instantaneously react to particular smells in very extreme ways. One woman told me when she was pregnant she became hypersensitive to the smell of newspaper print, something most of us cannot even detect, yet it would make her immediately feel nauseous and bring on debilitating migraines. Her husband did not believe her and he took to hiding his newspaper in their house. One day she came home and as soon as she opened the front door she could smell newspaper print. Eventually she found it carefully concealed in the cellar.

Another reason that makes it so difficult to design an olfactory space is that the senses of smell and taste are intertwined, thereby making it a particularly challenging task to try to consider smell in isolation. We have been conditioned to consider smell in conjunction with other sense activities, which often results in us neglecting to think about smell in its own right. I first started to think about smell in isolation when I was team teaching with a teacher who was blind. Every morning when we met we would have a prolonged conversation about smell. Over time I found myself developing a much more sophisticated ability to think about smell in isolation. It was the consistent, ongoing attention she gave to the sense of smell that helped to stimulate my interest. This is what the caring practitioner needs to do.

A third reason for the difficulty in designing an olfactory space relates to the kinds of problems children and adults experience with the olfactory sense. These problems can be so diverse, so extreme and, in the case of children and adults with learning difficulties, so tricky for the practitioner to observe and identify, that it is possible the practitioner may make serious olfactory errors without even being aware of them. Conditions related to smell that the practitioner needs to be aware of include: anosmia the total inability to smell, hyposmia a decreased ability to smell, hyperosmia an abnormally acute ability to smell, Olfactory Reference Syndrome where the person imagines they have a strong body odour, phantosmia where the person smells false odours particularly unpleasant ones, dysosmia where the person mismatches smells, parosmia where the person finds smells more unpleasant than most other people, and cacosmia where the person thinks things smell like faeces. The practitioner needs to be aware when designing an olfactory area that all these conditions are likely to be much more prevalent in children and adults with learning difficulties.

A fourth reason for the difficulty is the abundance of misinformation about the olfactory sense, especially in relation to aromatherapy. Practitioners must be especially careful with the way they provide olfactory stimulation and make certain they have a clear understanding of how the person is experiencing each smell activity. The biggest challenge is how to design the olfactory sense experience so it can be: controlled by the participant and only be made available when the participant wishes to partake in the experience, provided in ways where the odour is presented for an extremely brief duration but to be extended as required, and delivered in an extremely mild intensity and then increased as necessary. The initial pure prototype design of the olfactory space would therefore consist of a set of enclosed containers that have a tube that can be brought to the nose for smelling and a control where the intensity of the odour can be expertly modulated or abruptly terminated.

Interoception space

I placed the interoception space second because as we learnt in Chapter 2 much of the brain's energy goes into interoception. Furthermore the nervous system largely keeps the information provided by interoception at an unconscious level. This means we tend to inaccurately think of the senses of exteroception as being of far greater importance.

Interoception refers to senses that access stimuli from within the body to inform us about the body and its position in space. The interoception space is an area that focuses on providing stimulation to these senses. The vestibular system specialises in spatial orientation and balance while proprioceptors inform the individual about position, tension and movement of body parts. The muscle spindles specialise in changes in muscle length while the Golgi tendon organs specialise in changes in muscle tension.

In addition to regular practitioners, the interoception space is used by physiotherapists, occupational therapists and by specialist physical education teachers. Practitioners may use the room for leisure and recreation, for therapy and for education. Equipment that provides introceptive stimulation includes rockers, water bed, ball pool, swings of various shapes and sizes, therapy balls, balance beam, balance aids, scooter boards, spinning apparatus, walkers, standers, climbing equipment, exercise equipment, vibration exerciser, blocks, tunnels, obstacle equipment and ladders. Other activities are massage and joint range movements.

White room

The white room is the most common prototype used in dedicated spaces for multisensory stimulation. In its pure form it is a vehicle for stimulation through the visual sense. The entire room is painted white. The white ceiling, walls, windows and floor form a giant 3D screen on which roving visual effects can be projected. From a gestalt perspective the white room forms the ground while the light show becomes the figure. The constantly changing visual effects are achieved by a pin spot focused on a rotating mirror ball and/or by a wheel effects projector. Mirrors can multiply the effect. The room appeals to people with many different types of sense difficulties including those with cortical visual impairment. The overall white effect can be maintained by adding white furnishings, white curtains and equipment. Practitioners may use the room for leisure and recreation, for therapy and for education.

Dark room

The dark room, with its black ceiling, walls, windows and floor, forms a strong black ground on which objects are located with maximum definition and minimum distraction. The principal use of the dark room is for visual stimulation, both ophthalmic and cortical. Specialist equipment includes spot lights, colour slides, fibre optic spray, coloured and ultraviolet lights, pen light torches (flash lights), iridescent paint and play dough, iridescent or white gloves, iridescent or white puppets, iridescent or white construction blocks. Dark room equipment enables people with very low vision to actively engage in visual activities that would not be possible in other environments. Visual activities can be conducted to encourage visual detection, recognition, differentiation, tracking, crossing the midline, and hand–eye coordination pursuits such as painting, sculpture, puppet-play and construction games. Practitioners may use the room for leisure and recreation, for therapy and for education.

Grey room

The grey room is specifically designed so that the practitioner can use a low sensory arousal approach. The grey room has a uniform grey ceiling, walls and carpeted floor. Grey curtains obscure windows and grey dustcovers hide equipment and materials not currently in use. These measures reduce or eliminate extraneous stimuli and help prevent the participant from being distracted from the single activity he or she is to work on. A low arousal approach is used with participants who are experiencing too much arousal, such as participants with fetal alcohol syndrome and a range of related conditions that include problems with impulse control, recognising boundaries and executive functioning. In the grey room single stimulus effects are presented within a context of minimum distraction and maximum scaffolding for learning. A low sensory arousal approach helps to give greater prominence to the caring practitioner who gently but firmly guides the participant's engagement. Practitioners may use the room for leisure and recreation, for therapy and for education.

Acoustically sharp sound space

McLuhan (1961) reasoned that for many non-literate societies hearing was their major sense, not vision. According to Ong (1969, p. 634) such societies did not have a world 'view' per se, rather their socio-cultural experience consisted of a series of auditory events. The acoustically sharp sound space enables the practitioner to control and manipulate sounds in ways that punctuate these auditory events so as to maximise listening pleasure and engagement. Regardless as to whether vision or hearing is the dominant sense, research tells us that hearing plays a profound role in our emotional and mental health. Hearing is a tremendously important sense and the acoustically sharp sound space is suitable for all participants who would benefit from engaging in listening activities.

Blackout facilities enable vision to be removed at will and soundproofing ensures the space is not contaminated by extraneous noises. Wooden ceiling, walls and a sprung wooden floor help to acoustically sharpen sounds produced within the room, thereby making it the optimal space for hearing enjoyment and auditory stimulation. Oliver Sacks (2005, p. 27) quotes John Hull and his experience of hearing:

> Thus he speaks of how the sound of rain, never before accorded much attention, can now delineate a whole landscape for him, for its sound on the garden path is different from its sound as it drums on the lawn, or on the bushes in his garden, or on the fence dividing it from the road. 'Rain' he writes, 'has a way of bringing out the contours of everything; it throws a coloured blanket over previously invisible things'.

The principal use of the acoustically sharp sound space, however, is for those with hearing impairment, both auricular and cortical, including those with cochlear implants. In this sound space sounds can be presented in isolation or in combination, produced by self or by others and further emphasised by particular equipment such as a resonance board or musical instruments especially percussion. Sound differentiation is achieved by minimising the auditory ground while intensifying the auditory figure in ways that appeal to the participant. The space can also help the participant make personal auditory cause–effect connections. The practitioner adjusts the figure–ground relationship to suit the participant's auditory skills, interests and abilities, thereby making the room valuable for auditory training. Practitioners may use the room for leisure and recreation, for therapy and for education.

Acoustically dull sound space

A room becomes acoustically dull through the use of sound absorption techniques such as fabric-covered panels, carpets, curtains and placing felt under noise-making machines. Extraneous external sounds associated with the space such as fans, air conditioning or heating are reduced as much as possible through a combination of passive noise control methods (soundproofing), active noise control methods (sound masking devices such as a white noise machine) and noise cancellation devices (headphones).

This space is valuable for people who experience auditory-defensiveness, that is, they have such an excessive sensitivity to sound that they find common sounds painful and disorientating. This makes it very difficult for them to function in many external environments. The acoustically dull sound space provides the caring practitioner with maximum control of the introduction of sound thereby providing the participant with the opportunity to gradually experiment with sound in ways they can manage.

Tactile space

The tactile space is the design prototype dedicated to the experience of touch. My first experience of a serious tactile space occurred when a student of mine who was himself totally blind, and his two parents who were also totally blind, invited me to their place for dinner. When I arrived their house was in complete darkness and it remained that way for the entire evening. It was a tremendously exciting dinner party because my hosts were so adept at orienting themselves in the space and I was so amateur. I realised they were carefully observing me to determine whether I had the know-how to be their son's teacher so I had to quickly work out how to perform in independent, sophisticated ways relying predominately on my sense of touch.

The tactual and cutaneous senses, also known as the somatic senses, comprise a number of distinctly discrete skills such as touch (tactition), pressure, temperature and pain, which combine to produce even more refined capabilities. I think of it as a sense spiral, the further up the spiral you go, the more sophisticated the skills become. For example passive touch is vastly different to active touch, otherwise called haptic perception. This is because active touch involves the alliance of somatosensory perception and proprioception. For people who are blind, active touch can provide them with extraordinary ways of perceiving the world as evidenced by the blind biologist Geerat Vermeij who used touch to identify entirely new species of mollusc (Sacks 2005).

The tactile space has its own tactile logic. This means the space is made up of tactile features that relate to: texture (rough to smooth), density (hard to soft), state (gas to fluid to solid), surface to depth, size (small to large), temperature (hot to cold), vibration (static, gentle, vigorous) and shape.

Gustatory space

The gustatory space can be any place where food is served, however it is more a time that is set aside for the explicit engagement with taste sensations rather than a particular place. This could be during meal times or it could be during a therapy session. The important point about the gustatory space though is that it follows a gustatory paradigm. The space is all about taste experiences: taste detection, recognition, awareness, taste attending, locating particular tastes, making taste comparisons and developing an understanding of taste.

A gustatory space is particularly relevant for participants who may experience difficulties making gustatory discriminations such as what is safe to eat, knowing how much to eat and when to stop eating. It is also relevant for participants who experience gustatory defensiveness. Gustatory defensiveness involves an extreme sensitivity to flavour and texture coupled with an inability to be able to regulate those taste experiences. Problems with an inability to regulate taste experiences and gustatory defensiveness can result in an ongoing narrowing of the range of foods that might be consumed, a reduction in eating enjoyment and even lead to life-threatening malnutrition.

Interactive area

The interactive area is for participants who experience extreme difficulties with movement. It is a space where the participant is provided with opportunities to be active rather than passive. An understanding of the relationship between cause and effect is promoted through the use of switches or other devices that are easy to manipulate and have exaggerated rewards. Vocal-sensitive and/or movement-sensitive switches enable a participant to immediately and consistently produce a grand effect that is both rewarding and meaningful for that person. The goal of the interactive area therefore is to engender in the participant a sense of personal agency, to give participants an understanding that they are able to make positive changes in their lives. This is considered to be particularly important for people who spend much of their lives being done to – being fed, being cleaned, being transported from one location to another. Switches are designed to suit the ability of individual participants. They include large or small touch pads that can be manipulated by toes, feet, fingers, hands, arms or legs. Manipulation may range from gentle touch to squeeze, they may involve the use of levers, collar switches, even remote control. Multisensory rewards are determined by the imagination of the practitioner: tactile – fans, auditory – music, visual – lights, smell – aroma, taste – food/drink, and interactive – computer games.

Water area

The water area consists of a pool filled with water. The water area is used for proprioceptive stimulation, both static and dynamic. The water (the ground) provides a support for the participant's body (figure), and frees the participant to move in ways not normally possible outside the water (figure–ground relationship). This is because the water supports the participant's body and provides greater resistance when the participant is moving his or her limbs. The water area can be used with a wide range of participants with debilitating sensory conditions including: participants who are non-ambulatory, those with cerebral palsy or who have osteoarthritis. Warm water is generally soothing for people with painful skeletal conditions while a spa option can provide gentle to vigorous massage. Moving in water is good exercise and helps participants develop and maintain body concept, image and awareness. Effects of aqua therapy are cited as being good for body function, movement, balance, body strength, gait and wellbeing. Supplementary equipment, such as a jacuzzi, shower, waterfall, slide, lights and heating, increases the range of stimulation/activity choices that can be provided. Safety in water areas needs to be specifically addressed, both in staff members and training and also in maintaining the water free of contamination.

Soft play

The soft play environment is an enclosed space with padded ceiling, walls and play furniture. Participants, particularly children, use the space to explore, interact with equipment and each other, construct, manipulate objects, experiment, climb, jump, roll, slide, crawl and hide. The soft play environment provides a safe place where participants can take risks without fear of getting hurt. It is particularly suitable for young children with vision impairment, those with physical disability who are reluctant to play in a regular, less forgiving playground environment or children who are fearful. By creating a safe, secure environment (ground) the participant is able to take risks (figure) with a reduced fear of getting hurt (figure–ground relationship). The floor plan may consist of a multi-level set of platforms connected by steps and ramps. Play furniture consists of large, soft, solid shapes (cubes, pyramids, cones, tubes and wedges) made from nylon reinforced, flame retardant, lead free, PVC filled with fire resistant foam rubber and held in place with Velcro strips. Additional equipment may include hard plastic moulded shapes to form building blocks and playground equipment, a ball pool, an innerspring mattress or a trampoline.

Portable environment

The portable environment is a small environment (approximately one to two metres square) that can be folded up and stored in a container for easy transportation from one location to another. The portable environment is suitable for children of all ages and for home use by parents or caregivers. A simple example of a portable environment is a lamb's wool skin. The lamb's wool skin might be moved from the cot to the pram to the floor thereby ensuring constancy when the baby first starts to explore environments other than the cot, so in effect it is a transportable comfort zone. The portable environment may be built on a strong cloth base with multisensory features attached using Velcro. This means items can be easily removed for cleaning and ensures that they are kept in a stable location in relation to the child. The portable environment may include a range of multisensory stimulation features (visual, auditory, olfactory), graded in complexity from very simple to challenging. The advantage of this design prototype is that it can be made accessible to children who live in isolated and remote areas. Portable environments can be loaned from toy libraries and resource centres.

Virtual environment

The goal of virtual reality is to simulate stimulation to the sense organs to match what would be available in another environment. It is achieved in a variety of ways particularly through audio-visuals on surround 3D screens, computers or head mounted displays, and hand or body gloves to replicate movement. There are also some developments in the tactile area for people who are blind. Providing the person is able to function at a basic sensory level, virtual reality has the potential to enable the more capable person with disabilities to engage in activities that would otherwise be impossible. Examples of use of virtual environments include people with autism congregating on Brigadoon Island in Second Life, and those with cerebral palsy and speech disorders having avatars that travel and communicate in non-disabled ways (Bennett 2011). Virtual environments can be individualised to suit particular needs and this can give the person much greater control over an environment. Virtual environments are being used for nurorehabilitation, for teaching a person how to use a wheelchair, and to teach executive function for people with learning difficulties or those with agoraphobia how to prepare for travel by public transport.

Inclusive area

The inclusive area is a regular environment, such as a verandah, garden or playground, but heavily enriched with features that promote multisensory stimulation. The result is a space more suitable for those with disabilities, but strongly appealing to all children. The principal use of this design prototype is to promote inclusion in the mainstream. When regular schools accept students with disabilities in their school they have a legal responsibility to ensure that the school environment is inclusive, so that it is able to be used by the child with that particular disability in ways that are similar or that parallel those uses made by non-disabled children.

Pluralist environment

The pluralist environment promotes awareness and a multi-perspective understanding. It focuses on change of the dedicated space for multisensory stimulation over time. If the space stays the same it becomes stale and both participants and staff lose interest. Ideas to help make pluralist changes relate to the use of themes (such as the sea, space, festivals, Indigenous culture) and performances (such as art exhibitions, music, acting out a story) with value placed on diversity.

Social space

This design prototype is different to the other prototypes because it is focuses on social group interaction with peers, whereas the other prototypes focus on individualised, multisensory spaces. The social space helps the child develop a sense of 'who am I?', an essential prerequisite for communication and social interaction. It is a space for get-togethers:

> If parents and non-disabled brothers and sisters [and friends] see the children happy, laughing and relaxed, as they so often are in the . . . [dedicated space

for multisensory stimulation], they're going to relate to them more than if they see them cranky, throwing their arms and legs around, dribbling and angry.

(Therapist cited in Pagliano 1999, p. 10)

The principal use of this area is to promote a sense of self through communication in a sympathetic environment.

The hybrid multisensory environment

The design of the hybrid multisensory environment subsumes a wide range of different sensory paradigms with each paradigm being internally consistent. The goal is to enable the caring practitioner to design a space to suit the unique needs of a particular participant and then to re-design the same space to suit the next participant, even when the next participant's needs are vastly different. The design of the space dedicated to multisensory stimulation is limited only by the design team's imagination. However the final product need not be expensive. This is because with slow design, accessing local resources and recycling are desirable objectives.

Part II

A unified approach

Practitioners who use multisensory stimulation in their work with participants come from many different disciplines. These disciplines include, but are not restricted to: social care, occupational therapy, physiotherapy, communication therapy, diversional therapy, education, nursing, psychology, psychiatry and palliative care. As a result, approaches that use multisensory stimulation tend to vary, and can indeed differ widely, according to the discipline background of the practitioner. This is occurring even though the daily concerns of practitioners with regard to the participant are remarkably similar.

In Part II I present a unified approach for using multisensory stimulation for adoption by practitioners from any discipline background. It is hoped this unified approach will support the development of standards that stretch past particular discipline boundaries, facilitate greater transdisciplinary collaboration amongst professionals and promote more rigorous research. The unified approach is built on the ideas elaborated so far in this book to guide a sensory understanding of the issues and to direct the tenor of interventions.

If regular interaction in an everyday environment stimulates appropriate levels of sense-learning development, then targeted multisensory stimulation is not required. A unified approach is only necessary when the usual course of sense learning development has proven to be unsuccessful and, as a consequence, the child or adult is experiencing sensory-related learning difficulties, which result in sensory deprivation. Sensory deprivation causes severe disturbances in physical development, social and emotional functioning, behaviour and communication and learning.

In the unified approach, the fundamental premise for interventions is that the participant, the practitioner and the environment are all indispensable and they work together in extending the multisensory confines of the participant. In the unified approach, the multisensory focus is primary and the discipline-specific techniques used in interventions (though important) are secondary.

A unified approach takes into account the participant's willingness to partake in the activity, the practitioner–participant relationship and the target and goal of the multisensory stimulation, which are in turn further predicated on appropriate assessment and the application of relevant research. The key point is that targeted multisensory stimulation becomes the form of communication between the participant and the caring professional. This underlies why all three aspects, the participant, the controlled multisensory environment and the practitioner, are so essential.

To reinforce this point, we have already learnt in previous chapters that when the multisensory stimulation is accessible, demand-free, choice-driven, empowering, meaningful and pleasurable to the user, it becomes a medium for communication, something the participant shares with the practitioner. If the practitioner does not notice and appreciate this sharing then the all-important precise confirmation does not occur. Confirmation is essential to help the participant identify a better self, to make a transition into a higher stage of development.

Once communication has been established then it may be used to support different applications of multisensory stimulation including play, leisure and recreation, therapy and education. Each specialist practitioner brings their own understanding of the issues involved, both from theoretical standpoints within their own discipline and from practical expertise derived from a pool of evidence-based practice regarding the way multisensory stimulation is used.

Part II is organised around the six essential stages underpinning the unified approach. These are:

1   Establishing a caring relationship (Chapter 7).
2   Assessment (Chapter 8).
3   Redesigning the environment (Chapter 9).
4   Beginning a sensory conversation (Chapter 10).
5   Extending the conversation (Chapter 11).
6   Catching the wave (Chapter 12).

Establishing a caring relationship

Introduction

The unified approach must begin with the practitioner establishing a caring relationship with the participant. This relationship is essential for the practitioner to be able to use multisensory stimulation to effectively communicate with the participant and for the participant to be able to effectively communicate with the practitioner. Establishing a caring relationship is much more complicated than it initially appears. This is because it involves considerable preparation and it requires a very substantial skill set.

Even though this relationship is the essential first step, sadly it is an area where there are many serious problems, particularly if the participant has difficulties with communication. One major issue is the tendency of the practitioner to take the relationship for granted. The practitioner often just assumes a good relationship has been established and he or she fails to check regularly for confirming and disconfirming evidence from the participant. This is usually compounded by lack of genuine reflection by the practitioner on his or her practice and by the practitioner's failure to closely examine his or her assumptions regarding people with disabilities in general and the participant in particular. Lack of reflection leaves considerable room for ongoing self-delusion.

As Jean Luc, the father of a girl with profound, multiple disabilities confides:

> My daughter Amélie must trust the practitioner before she will engage. This trust comes from the practitioner developing a caring relationship with her. If practitioners do not have a caring relationship it is because of their assumptions: their prejudices, their stereotypes, and their problems with discrimination towards people with multiple disabilities and disorders of communication. It has nothing to do with Amélie!

As we have already learnt in Chapter 4, if the participant does not trust the professional then the participant will not be willing to engage in novel activities, so no progress can be made. Without establishing a caring relationship and assiduously maintaining that relationship, the unified approach cannot continue.

So what sorts of assumptions get in the way of the practitioner establishing a caring relationship? To help answer that question I want to share a story. Sue, a friend of mine, works in an institution that has a controlled multisensory environment room for people with disabilities. This room was rented out every week for one afternoon session to two adults with profound disabilities and significant disorders of communication. Usually Sue did not have anything to do with the way the room was used during these sessions. However one day she was in the storeroom putting things away when she inadvertently observed through the mirror window the two participants being led into the room by their two assistants.

The two assistants made no attempt to communicate with the participants. One participant was swiftly deposited onto the waterbed and the other was just as rapidly plonked in front of a bubble tube. The two assistants then withdrew from the participants and threw themselves into the ball pool. Sue thought this indicated it was a regular practice. The assistants then proceeded to spend the entire session loudly chatting to each other about their boyfriends and sending text messages on their mobile phones. At no time did they interact with their charges. At no time did they check whether the participants were engaging with the equipment or even discuss how they were faring. As far as the assistants were concerned, the multisensory environment was the activity so their input was not required. The assistants were free to do whatever they liked.

After the session Sue said she assertively tried to engage the two assistants in a conversation but they were dismissive. It suited the assistants to think the multisensory environment was a self-contained beneficial entity. This meant it was not their responsibility to do anything. As far as Sue could ascertain the two participants did not engage with any of the activities in the room. Instead the participants seemed to be disengaged and one started to vigorously slap her own head. Sue told me later that she felt the whole experience was a complete waste of time for all and, even worse, detrimental to the participants' wellbeing. Yet it was an activity the four of them attended regularly one afternoon each week and no doubt the assistants were being paid to be there. Sue reported that even when she tried to challenge the assistants to reflect on their relationship with their participants they simply said: 'Oh we've got great relationships. We love them and they love us. They're our friends.'

Contrary to their protestations, the evidence would indicate that while the assistants were in the multisensory environment they did not establish nor did they maintain a caring relationship with their participants. According to Noddings what makes the relationship a caring relationship is recognition on the part of the cared-for that an act of caring has taken place. That is what Jean Luc was referring to. It is this recognition in the cared-for that establishes the foundation for trust, and initiates willingness on the part of the participant to take risks and to try to communicate, to make meaning. This caring relationship is established through a process of engrossment, an ongoing absorption in the cared-for. The carer is as open as possible to what the cared-for is trying to communicate. The greater the cared-for's difficulty with communication, the more engrossed the carer must become to be able to decipher the cared-for's intentions.

This caring relationship is based on a set of principles regarding how a caring practitioner ought to behave when working with a participant, particularly someone who is vulnerable. These principles unambiguously and consistently guide the provision of high quality care. The care value base requires the practitioner to ensure their assumptions and practices are not prejudicial, stereotyped or discriminatory.

Prejudice involves making judgements about a person before sufficient information is obtained to ensure accuracy. The best way for a practitioner to avoid behaving in prejudicial ways is to keep ongoing records and to hold off making judgements until after assessment has been conducted. Prejudice is sometimes confused with stereotype and they often go hand in hand but the two terms are different.

A stereotype is an understanding or judgement that does not change over time. For example a practitioner may make the assumption that he or she will observe the same behaviours in all people with a particular condition. This stereotype may then influence the way that person interacts with a new participant. The best way for a practitioner to avoid stereotypes is to treat each person as an individual and to make careful note of changes that occur in the participant over time.

Discrimination refers to the act of excluding or restricting individuals because of their membership of a particular group. Not having wheelchair access to a building therefore would be discriminatory against people who require such access. There are many examples in the literature of people with disorders of communication being discriminated against because they do not literally have a voice with which to express their concerns. The whole idea of establishing a caring relationship is to help prevent discrimination occurring.

The core value base of any practitioner who works in a helping profession is very similar and that helps the unified approach. The core value base for those practitioners working with a participant with a sensory disability using targeted multisensory stimulation focuses on questions relating to how to behave in ethical ways, how to protect the rights of the participant and how best to work with the participant when in the multisensory environment. Specific core values discussed below are: build on the relationship, mindfulness, beneficence and non-maleficence, employ a non-pathologising approach, work with the participant, design approaches for empowerment, go deep, recognise treatment may be flawed, and acknowledge that sometimes it might not be possible to help. Given that each value is an essential, integrated part of establishing a caring relationship, the order of presentation is necessarily somewhat arbitrary.

Build on the relationship

As already stated the practitioner starts by establishing a caring relationship and continues to assiduously work to maintain it. The practitioner builds on the caring relationship by basing it on congruence, trust, empathy and unconditional positive regard (Rogers 1957). I will discuss congruence and trust first and then examine empathy and unconditional positive regard under the next heading, mindfulness.

For a relationship to be congruent it must be authentic. Congruence is the single most important attribute of a caring relationship. If the practitioner is not genuine then he or she should not continue to work in the field. The reason congruence is so central is the sincerity must be extended or modelled to the participant to help the participant achieve greater congruence in his or her own life. That is how the practitioner in a caring relationship uses confirmation to help the participant achieve a better self, to reduce the incongruence between the participant's current self and the participant's potential self.

A by-product of a caring relationship is the development of trust. This trust must be strictly nurtured and protected. At all times the participant must feel safe and secure with the practitioner and safe and secure with the activities being offered. The caring relationship is the envelope through which the interaction occurs. If the envelope is damaged then the participant might not accept the message.

Through trust a special participant–practitioner relationship emerges. This trust means the practitioner has power over the participant, and the use of this power must be informed by ethical guidelines, in particular the practitioner's attention to boundaries. For example the practitioner is friendly to the participant but not their friend. This is a critical point because in a friendship there is the mutual opening up of self, whereas in the practitioner–participant relationship the focus is on helping the participant. The relationship is not equal so it is not a friendship relationship and it is inaccurate to call it one.

When establishing the relationship the practitioner must simultaneously pay close attention to five key boundary perspectives. They are: propriety, space, behavioural, verbal/non-verbal, energy and somatic. These are discussed below.

Propriety refers to the level of respect that must be attributed to the participant. This respect is informed by basic human rights (see United Nations 2011). Even when the participant exhibits extreme challenging behaviour the practitioner must maintain a high level of decorum as befits a professional. Sometimes this is difficult, such as when a participant suddenly and unexpectedly strongly punches you in the back during a session. Fortunately the other boundaries help you to guard against such an incident occurring.

Spatial boundaries refer to the physical distance between the practitioner and the participant necessary for mutual comfort and for effective treatment. These spatial boundaries are also important for your own self-protection. You need to feel safe too! Trust is a two-way street. Be aware that complications with proximity can occur particularly if the participant has certain aberrant behaviours (see discussion of stereotypy in Chapter 8, p. 103). These conditions and behaviours may preclude close contact. When working with participants with challenging behaviour you may need to take more time to ensure that the participant feels sufficiently comfortable before beginning an activity. Sometimes the practitioner may simply need to ask the participant if they feel comfortable with their physical arrangement, and then adjust accordingly. Other times the practitioner must read between the lines to work out a suitable and mutually safe working distance. A perceptive practitioner will use ongoing non-verbal indicators to ensure the participant always has adequate personal space.

Behavioural boundaries refer to the need for both the practitioner and the participant to address personal needs. For example on occasions the practitioner might need to reschedule a session or cut it short if he or she does not feel well or there is a family emergency. The practitioner must also take into account how the participant is feeling. If the participant is not well then the activities will need to be adjusted accordingly. Behavioural boundaries are a product of emotional self-regulation so they are there for protection. For example with empathy the practitioner tries to understand the participant's situation and reflect it back to the participant without over-identifying with it. Similarly when the participant engages in challenging behaviour the practitioner works to maintain a sense of self rather than be carried away by the situation.

Verbal and non-verbal boundaries come from being in contact with and understanding yourself, what you can effectively manage and what is too difficult for you. The practitioner needs to be aware of what is right for the moment and be sufficiently comfortable to clearly state preferences such as 'I like . . . I do not like . . .'. Practitioners who do not clearly establish verbal and non-verbal boundaries risk developing compassion fatigue. For example a practitioner might be negatively affected by certain smells that occur when the participant has toileting problems. If the practitioner has difficulties with these, then be up-front and deal with them rather than taking on a martyr role.

Understanding energy and somatic boundaries are particularly important when more intimate treatments are being used such as massage. Here the practitioner must explicitly establish his or her own boundaries and constantly check that the participant feels comfortable in the process. Remember the participant may choose to end a treatment at any time without providing a reason.

Mindfulness

Mindfulness is similar to engrossment. Noddings described engrossment as a state of continuing complete absorption, whereas mindfulness involves giving one's best attention and empathy. Empathy is the ability to be able to unsympathetically recognise and even sensitively and accurately share another person's experiences and feelings. By unsympathetic I mean neither approving nor not approving. The experience of empathy in the practitioner engenders a desire to help the participant.

Empathy starts as an affective response where judgement is suspended to better understand the participant's experiences and progresses to a cognitive response where this understanding is reflected back to the participant in a professional way. An important part of empathy is this ability to maintain an unconditional positive regard for the participant. This enables the practitioner to approve of the participant even if they do not approve of the participant's behaviour. The special kind of attention therefore is open, non-judgemental and purposeful.

We have already discussed the need for engrossment (see Chapter 5) in order to more precisely gauge what the participant is actually experiencing sense-wise. Mindfulness is useful because it provides the practitioner with more explicit information about how to purposefully engage in engrossment. Greason and Cashwell (2009) describe four aspects of mindfulness attention that are available to the practitioner. They are:

1 Selective attention. This is where the practitioner foregrounds some things while backgrounding others. The practitioner sorts information into what is most relevant and important in the here and now and what is not. To be able to apply selective attention, the practitioner needs to have an advanced metacognitive understanding of the situation. Metacognition is sometimes defined as knowing about knowing. Not only does the practitioner need to understand the big picture, but he or she must also be able to play with that understanding in controlled ways. Much of what I have been writing in this book is aimed at helping the practitioner gain this know-how. The practitioner works from a big picture perspective and then zeros in to follow lines of observation that check whether certain predictions are accurate or not. For example if the practitioner was trying to gauge whether the participant could detect a visual stimulus, the practitioner would be foregrounding the way the participant's eyes were behaving and closely observing facial expressions for particular clues, while backgrounding all other information.

2 Divided attention. This is where the practitioner maintains concentration on more than one thing at a time. Divided attention is therefore an even more sophisticated mindfulness skill than selected attention. Divided attention is important for the practitioner to be able to maintain a caring relationship and do something with the attention. The practitioner focuses on the participant and what the participant is communicating (verbally/ non-verbally), while simultaneously conducting lines of enquiry. For example divided attention might be necessary if the participant starts to demonstrate discomfort during a line of enquiry. The divided attention may be necessary to determine if the discomfort is related to the line of enquiry or whether it is due to some non-related factor such as the participant

wanting to go to the toilet or have a break. This is where timely communication comes into play. The practitioner checks with the participant regarding what to do next.

3   Sustained attention. This is where the practitioner maintains high levels of focused attention for extended periods of time. Sustained attention enables the practitioner to gain a much deeper and more accurate understanding of what the participant is experiencing. Sustained attention may be required when the practitioner is trying to observe whether the participant has achieved a transition, like moving from being able to recognise a stimulus to being able to make differentiations. Sustained attention is required when the practitioner is providing confirming feedback. The more precise the confirming feedback, the more powerful the message for the participant. Conversely, the less precise the confirming feedback, the less powerful the message for the participant.

4   Attention switching. This is where the practitioner rapidly jumps from one focal point area to another. Attention switching may be necessary if the practitioner has a number of concerns regarding the participant and needs to keep these concerns under observation. When a practitioner first starts to work with a participant, attention switching may be a useful way of collecting a wide range of different types of information about the participant.

These four aspects of attention and the empathy work together to create a synergy that becomes mindfulness.

Beneficence and non-maleficence

Beneficence is the idea of acting only to benefit the participant, while non-maleficence refers to doing no harm. Beneficence and non-maleficence together provide a key foundation for ethical practice. Beneficent actions include preventing and removing harmful factors whenever possible and only doing things that promote recuperation and/or wellbeing. As all handling of vulnerable people engenders some risk, the practitioner must at all times carefully balance benefits against risks and as much as possible explicitly involve the participant in the decision making process. The practitioner must invite the participant to go into the multisensory environment and wait for a positive response before proceeding. Furthermore, while in the room the participant helps to decide how long the activity will continue, when the activity is over and when to leave the room. To be better able to carefully balance benefits against risks the practitioner should take into account relevant evidence-based practice (EBP) and empirically-supported treatments (EST) and take particular care not to provide any treatment that has no possibility of benefit.

Employ a non-pathologising approach

Pathology is the scientific study of diseases and abnormal conditions so a pathological approach makes the central aim of the treatment the amelioration of the disease or condition. While a pathology-centred approach is an appropriate model for medical interventions, it is not so relevant to most of the disciplines that use multisensory stimulation in their work with participants. For these disciplines, it is important the practitioner treats the participant within their personal context, in other words caters to the needs of the whole person, particularly the person's socio-cultural background, temperament and personality, and involves the person in the decision making process. The participant is the focus, not the pathology.

Using a non-pathologising approach is especially the case when working with the participant in the multisensory environment. In the past some practitioners in the multisensory environment over-concentrated on the pathology to the neglect of the participant and treatments were much less effective because the participant was not an active part of the solution. One danger of a pathologising approach is that it leads to the practitioner adopting stereotypes, which, as we have already noted, can get in the way of establishing a caring relationship.

Two non-pathologising measures are: using non-categorical language and separating the person from the behaviour. Non-categorical language places the person first and the descriptor second, that is, 'person with a disability' not 'disabled person'. This person first, condition second, language reminds the participant and the practitioner that the treatment is for the whole person. Separating the person from the behaviour involves a similar reframing. Once the behaviour is separated from the participant the therapist can focus on two things: building and maintaining a positive relationship with the participant and designing a treatment to help decrease the problem behaviour.

For example 'angry participant' becomes a participant who experiences problems with anger at particular times and in particular circumstances. This new way of thinking about the situation helps the practitioner focus on the context of the behaviour and better understand probable causes, such as the participant becomes angry at feeding time, possibly because eating has become a painful activity.

Another example is if a participant suddenly punches me, my spontaneous reaction might be to think the participant hit me because he or she disliked me. After separating the behaviour from the participant and discussing the incident with the participant's family I might then realise the punching was a form of stereotypical behaviour, which had nothing to do with me per se.

Work with the participant

Hippocrates (BC 460–370), the father of modern medicine, stressed the importance of working with the natural healing forces of the body. A parallel idea continues to underpin all interactions in the multisensory environment today. The practitioner works with the participant's innate sensory framework to design activities congruent with participant needs, and whenever possible invites the participant to lead the process. The key to working with the participant's innate sensory framework is to use mindfulness to more accurately identify what the participant can already do and to then determine what is the natural next step.

The practitioner does this by closely observing the participant, listening to what the participant is saying verbally/non-verbally and through careful observation of the participant's general demeanour. The practitioner then uses his or her own professional expertise, experience and know-how to design activities that provide the participant with increased opportunities to meet these needs, for the participant to build on his or her own strengths in ways that are congruent with the natural sensory process. Working with the participant's innate sensory framework, building on strengths and involving the participant in the process helps increase the likelihood that the treatment will be more effective and long-lasting.

Design approaches for empowerment

A logical extension of the non-pathologising approach is a focus on the empowerment of the participant. For this to happen, the practitioner must first believe in the possibility that the participant's control over his or her own life can be expanded by an activity.

Empowerment is multidimensional: psychological (the way a participant thinks about him/herself), sociological (the way a participant relates to others) and political (the way power is used). Empowerment is a process because it occurs over time and involves development. In this process the participant takes greater control of his/her own life in ways important to the participant. This in turn makes the participant more self-sufficient, autonomous and independent. The process changes the practitioner–participant relationship. As the participant becomes more independent and the participant requires less assistance from the practitioner, a new relationship emerges, one in which the participant achieves greater levels of participation. So empowerment becomes a form of participatory action research, where the interaction is genuinely democratic and non-coercive.

Beatrice Wright (1960) argued that the language we use can either be empowering or devaluing. She warned about the pervasive dangers inherent in practitioners over focusing on the negatives regarding a person's condition, believing that over time these negatives lead to the practitioner adopting a negative bias. Wright also cautioned against the spread effect where it is assumed that a person with one disability also has other disabilities, for example thinking a person with a physical impairment also has an intellectual impairment, or the action of talking loudly to someone who is blind.

The idea that the structure of language affects the way we conceptualise the world is known as the Sapir–Whorf hypothesis (Hoijer 1954). In parallel with the Sapir–Whorf hypothesis, at an even more profound level, the way we use our senses to engage with the world strongly influences our conception of the world – this concept is central to this book.

Go deep

A goal of the unified approach is to go beyond the superficial focus on symptoms, to address how the person experiences meaning and purpose. This goal is particularly important when working with participants who experience profound difficulties with the senses. This is because early sense-learning development lays the foundation for meaning acquisition so the person may still be in the very early formative stages of finding meaning. The idea of going deep comes from the three Viennese schools of psychotherapy, those of Freud, Adler and Frankl.

We effectively looked at Freud's will to pleasure (Freud 1920) in Chapter 3 learning that pleasure is a state of being that involves the gratification of the senses. The pleasure derived from the sense experience provides the motivation for the person to continue to use the senses into the future. Success is a powerful motivator. A major concern for children and adults with profound, multiple disabilities is how little success they encounter in their daily life. Three different types of pleasure were introduced. Ease is associated with the primitive brain. It is a subconscious feeling of comfort and contentment. In-the-moment pleasure is a conscious enjoyment of a sense experience while it is actually occurring. Anticipatory pleasure is where the person looks forward to a repeat of in-the-moment experience. It is the interplay of these three pleasure types that stimulates sense-learning development.

Adler's will to power (Adler 1956) has also been influential in this book. Throughout this book I have consistently stressed the importance of equality between the practitioner and the participant and the need for the practitioner to think about a person in a holistic manner. According to Adler it is a person's will to power that makes it possible for the individual to change for the better. This idea led to the development of Maslow's hierarchy (see Chapter 6) and Noddings' confirmation of a better self (see Chapter 5). In Chapter 6 I talked about the need to apply user-centred design principles to ensure that the controlled multisensory environment could be designed and redesigned around the interests and abilities of the individual, thereby making power experiences more easily accessible.

The third Viennese school, that of Frankl (1946), focused on the will to meaning and purpose. This will to meaning was the main idea behind Chapter 5. In Chapter 5 the quest of the chapter was how to help the person achieve the ability to make meaning. Frankl maintained that the will to meaning is the individual's original pursuit. He said that it is only when the will to meaning is frustrated that a person allows themselves to become intoxicated with pleasure or power. Interesting Frankl argued that meaning is discovered in three ways: through experience, through creative action and through other people. The way we offer meaning to a person with profound multiple disabilities therefore involves providing opportunities for that individual to experience sensory stimulation, waiting for the experience to activate a desire in the person to make a creative response, and for a caring practitioner to reflect that response back to the person so that it can be interpreted in a meaningful way.

In interactions that focus on the idea of finding meaning and purpose the emphasis is less on being and more on becoming. The practitioner aims to help the participant find his or her own path towards self-awareness. It is a process of helping to set the participant free.

Recognise treatment may be flawed

No matter how high quality the treatment is, how scientifically well regarded it is, or how much EBP is available to support it, each time a treatment is provided the yardstick is how it is received by the participant. As a consequence the wise practitioner makes no assumptions and constantly checks and rechecks that the treatment is progressing satisfactorily and in the manner predicted. Practitioners have a number of tools at their disposal to monitor what is happening. These include conducting appropriate assessment at every stage, involving the participant in the process and consulting others to ensure that their observations are accurate. To achieve this practitioners use triangulation, a process of data validation through cross verification. Triangulation often involves the comparison of three different measures. Measures may differ by observer, time, location, theoretical stance or data gathering method.

Acknowledge that sometimes it might not be possible to help

Being a practitioner means we are limited and it is critical to acknowledge this limitation both to ourselves and to our participants. As practitioners we need to undertake our work with humility and to not make promises we cannot keep. No matter how much expertise and experience we have, sometimes the repertoire of activities we have at our disposal may not fit the needs of the participant, so we must adjust our expectations accordingly and be upfront about what we may or may not be able to achieve.

All our participants are exceptional. Their exceptionality may mean that you as a practitioner have never previously encountered a particular behavioural set. Some participants have deteriorating conditions where progress is not possible and the most that might be able to be achieved is an improvement in wellbeing. Despite this, it is essential for the practitioner to maintain a discipline of hope. Even though all we can do is our best, if our best is practised within a context of hope and genuine reflection this provides us with a greater likelihood that a breakthrough might be achieved. The practitioner therefore needs to balance reality with optimism and adjust activities accordingly. Transdisciplinary liaison can be invaluable.

Chapter 8

Assessment

Introduction

All assessment is anchored in the unified approach to using multisensory stimulation and its theoretical framework that has been developed throughout this book. Understanding this framework is a requirement to being able to clearly define assessment goals – which participants are to be assessed, what is to be assessed, how, when and by whom. The framework is based on four pillars, namely: wellbeing, development, learning and function (see Figure 8.1).

The unified approach is built on these four pillars because conducting assessment that focuses on just one area does not adequately cater to the exceptional

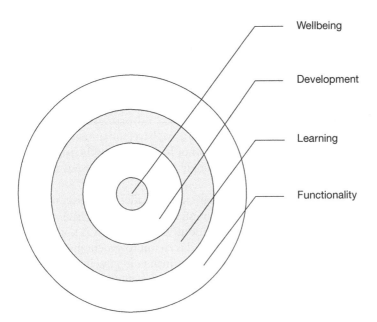

Figure 8.1 Four pillars of the unified approach to using multisensory stimulation.

needs of participants. For example, learning by itself is inadequate because it is based on an assumption of progress, which excludes participants with regressive conditions. Development by itself is also inadequate because wellbeing is an essential prerequisite for sense-learning development to take place. Finally function, the fourth pillar, is required to cater for participants who miss critical developmental stages because of their disabilities or their regressive conditions, but may still attain compensatory or adaptive behaviours that enable them to function more independently.

Assessment used in the unified approach covers five areas. These are: wellbeing, stereotypy, engagement, interoception and exteroception.

Conducting assessment on participants with sense-learning difficulties is challenging. Participants are likely to present with incomplete assessment information. Frequently participants will not have had up-to-date comprehensive medical, hearing, vision, dental nor other functional assessments such as in physiotherapy, occupational therapy and speech language pathology, nor will they have been prescribed prosthetic devices such as glasses, hearing aids and cochlear implants. What assessment information that does arrive from other services might be vague, dated or irrelevant to the unified approach where the focus in on the participant being able to make meaning out of multisensory stimulation and use this understanding to communicate with others. The practitioner may therefore need to start the assessment process from scratch.

When conducting assessment with participants with sense-learning difficulties it is essential to remember that the assessment only provides information about what a person can do at a particular point in time. It does not necessarily tell you about what the person cannot do. Also the participant's ability may fluctuate markedly, especially if the participant has significant other health problems. Assessment information needs to be always considered within the current context. It is a tool to inform practitioner practice with the participant.

When assessing participants with sensory learning difficulties the quality of the participant–practitioner relationship markedly influences the quality of the assessment. Before detailed assessment can even begin in earnest, the practitioner must have established a caring relationship with the participant. The participant must trust the practitioner and the environment.

When participants have very limited skills and abilities, options regarding objective assessment measures are limited. The practitioner therefore needs to rely much more heavily on his or her own expertise, observation abilities and insights. This requires careful validation.

In the unified approach there is a primary focus on the participant's sensory ability. This is because sense development is regarded as the gateway to all further development. The participant, the caring practitioner and the multisensory environment are an indissoluble trinity.

In assessment using the unified approach great attention is paid to the affective. The focus is on the expansion of the participant's sense abilities, to improve participant wellbeing, development, learning and functionality. Most caring practitioners come from a discipline background (usually education or therapy). Discipline considerations are important but secondary, being only a vehicle with which to achieve change.

Detailed observations of the participant's behaviour by the caring practitioner become an essential part of the assessment process. It is a dynamic process consisting of ongoing purposeful information gathering, analysis and reflection. As a result, decisions are made by the caring practitioner about the design of a multisensory programme targeted to engage and ultimately expand the sensory thresholds of the participant. The precise nature of the programme is discipline-dependent using unified approach principles. Intervention is followed by reassessment. The result is a spiral never-ending process whose success depends on the precision and expertise of the caring practitioner. It is not a 'one size fits all' approach.

Types of assessment

The following eight scopes of assessment measures (Neisworth and Bagnato 1988) and play assessment are relevant to participants with sense-learning difficulties and the unified approach. They can either be used by themselves or in conjunction with each other.

Ecological assessment: the goal of an ecological assessment is to describe the nature of interactions between the participant and his or her environment. The practitioner therefore collects evidence detailing the participant's development within a range of environments pertinent to the participant's life. Assessment may involve studying the participant's file to gain a historical perspective, interviewing major stakeholders associated with each environment, conducting on-location assessment and making unobtrusive observations within those environments. This type of assessment helps the practitioner using the unified approach to gain a broader understanding of sense ability functioning in each of the participant's principal environments.

Judgement-based assessment: judgement-based assessment comes to the fore when it is not possible to obtain high quality objective or subjective assessment information directly from the participant because of a lack of formal assessment instruments and/or the participant's inability to communicate. With judgement-based assessment the practitioner collects as much relevant information as possible, then structures it and integrates it in ways that enable the practitioner to make well-considered professional judgements about the participant's wellbeing and performance. Judgement-based assessment is strengthened when professionals from different disciplines cross-reference their judgements and use further assessment to check for confirming and disconfirming evidence. In the unified approach the focus of judgement-based assessment is on more precisely describing the participant's sense windows.

Process assessment: in this type of assessment, the practitioner concentrates on collecting information about the participant while in the controlled multisensory environment. The practitioner is particularly interested in obtaining information that details the process that is the series of minute facial, physical and behavioural changes that occur in the participant during the actual session. This kind of information is especially valuable when the participant has very limited ability to communicate. The minute changes help to inform the practitioner about the participant's wellbeing and current levels of sensory engagement. As it is extremely difficult for the practitioner to unreservedly concentrate on observing these micro changes and to simultaneously interpret them during the session, the practitioner may resort to the assistance of a specially trained observer, to making video recordings of the session, and to conducting collaborative reflection sessions where a team of experts gather to more deeply analyse the assessment information.

Interactive assessment: interactive assessment is similar to process assessment however here the centre of attention is on participant interaction with the sensory stimulation, the object, the person or the event. Interactive assessment is a particularly important form of assessment in the unified approach where so much significance is placed on the role of the caring professional and the relationship between the participant and the practitioner. As with process assessment, the practitioner obtains information detailing the minute facial, physical and behavioural changes that occur in the participant during the actual session; however now these are considered in the context of each participant interaction. A further similarity to process assessment is the practical difficulty the practitioner faces trying to make observations regarding interactions between him/herself and the participant and vice versa. It is therefore valuable for the practitioner to have the assistance of a specially trained observer, to make video recordings of the session, and to conduct collaborative reflection sessions with a team of experts.

Adaptive-to-handicap assessment: adaptive behaviour is any behaviour that contributes directly to a person's survival so it includes eating, drinking and communication. Adaptive-to-handicap assessment is therefore directed towards function. Many sense-learning difficulties have a significant impact on a person's ability to act independently. Adaptive-to-handicap assessment therefore identifies whether the participant is able to perform an equivalent behaviour through the assistance of specially designed environmental modifications and/or a different sense skill set. For example a head switch may enable a participant to turn on Christmas tree lights if his or her hands are not able to manage the task.

Curriculum-based assessment: with curriculum-based assessment a learning outcome is used to inform instruction and assessment is then conducted to verify whether the outcome has been achieved. If it has not been achieved then the instruction is adjusted accordingly. This type of assessment is used to measure student mastery of objectives within a continuum of objectives specified by a particular educational institution's schedule of learning. Curriculum-based assessment is an important education assessment tool, which comes more into focus once the participant has moved out of the unified approach and the practitioner has returned back to his or her own discipline, in this case education.

Norm-based assessment: the aim of this form of assessment is to compare the participant's developmental skills with those of the same-aged general population. Such information may not be particularly helpful when assessing participants who are substantially outside the norm; however it does provide the practitioner with potentially valuable information about where the participant is at developmentally and the likely developmental sequence to be followed.

Systematic observation: using highly structured surveillance methods to conduct assessment is particularly valuable in the controlled multisensory environment, especially when trying to assess a difficult-to-assess participant. This approach, which includes direct observation, checklists and video recording, helps to uncover many otherwise missed assessment opportunities. Ways to make the observations even more systematic involve: descriptive notes to clearly specify foreshadowed notions regarding what the participant might possibly be capable of achieving, creating a list of behaviour expectations, and developing benchmark indicators to guide your search for particular types of evidence. A benchmark indicator would be a description of behaviours that clearly and unambiguously demonstrate that a participant can actually perform a particular skill. These same indicators can also be used to form a continuum to chart behavioural approximations, that is behaviours that are in the direction of the benchmark but not quite there yet. The beauty of video recordings is that they can be used to establish a baseline and can be revisited at later dates. This information can then be shared with major stakeholders.

The disadvantage of video assessment is that it requires good lighting, which may compromise the environment.

A ninth form is play-based assessment, which is when the participant is formally observed at play. In play-based assessment the emphasis is on the participant being in control and the practitioner merely a facilitator. This fits well with the ethos of the multisensory environment. It is the participant who makes the rules and it is the practitioner's responsibility to ensure that he or she provides guidance that is built on a well established, mutually trusting and respectful relationship with the participant.

First steps

The first thing you will need to do once you have accepted a new participant is to conduct an initial interview with the key stakeholders. Key stakeholders are all those who perceive themselves to have a major caring role in the life of the participant. They are usually the recognised carer(s) of the person with the sense disability. For people living in institutions, however, there might not be a single carer, rather there may be several people with more minor roles. It is still worthwhile involving these people in the initial interview if this is possible.

The initial interview follows a semi-structured format where the practitioner requests basic demographic information such as name, age, gender, address, contact details, family/social details, services received details, medical details as well as information about personal likes and dislikes and communication styles (see Table 8.1).

Table 8.1 Initial interview template

(Modify items on this template to suit your information needs)
Name of participant: _____
Person conducting the interview: _____
Date interview completed: _____

Gender of participant (state name): M/F
Date of birth: _____
Name(s) of people being interviewed: _____
Relationship to participant (state name): _____
Relevant address(es): _____
Contact details: _____
Telephone: _____
Mobile: _____
Email: _____
Fax: _____

Family/social
Who lives with the participant (state name)? _____
Who often sees the participant (state name)? _____
Who occasionally sees the participant (state name)? _____
Draw the participant's (state name) family tree showing
extended and blended family, ages, occupations, significant attributes:
_____
_____
_____

Who are the most important figures in the participant's (state name) life?
_____

What are the most important places in the participant's (state name) life?
_____

What have been the most important events in the participant's (state
name) life? _____

Services received
What services does the participant (state name) currently receive?
Give full details: _____
Who are the participant's (state name) doctor(s)? _____
Contact details: _____
Who are the participant's (state name) therapist(s)? _____
Contact details: _____
List other relevant services received: _____

Continued

Continued

Medical history
When did you first know there were problems? _____
What happened then? (Attach sheet if necessary) _____

Checklist – medical

_____ ❑ Birth details (if relevant)
_____ ❑ Vaccinations
_____ ❑ Serious illnesses
_____ ❑ Operations
_____ ❑ Medications
_____ ❑ Allergies

The participant
Tell me about the participant's (state name) interests, likes and dislikes:
_____
_____
_____
_____
_____

Comment on the participant's (state name) current status with regard to the following:

Sensorimotor status
Balance   _____
Smell   _____
Taste   _____
Touch   _____
Hearing   _____
Vision   _____
Other   _____

Communication
How does the participant (state name) communicate the following?

Yes   _____
No   _____
Drink   _____
Toilet _____
Happy   _____
Sad   _____
Other   _____

What are your hopes, fears, concerns for the participant (state name), both now and in the long term?

_____

_____

_____

_____

_____

Other issues:

_____

_____

_____

_____

Other relevant information:

_____

_____

_____

_____

Signature: _____

The initial interview is not just an opportunity to gather valuable background information, it is also an opportunity to start to develop a two-way relationship with the key stakeholder. The template provides an opening for the key stakeholder to offer a detailed snapshot of how he/she perceives the participant's current sensorimotor status and for the voicing of hopes, fears and expectations regarding the participant. The more complete and insightful the information you are able to obtain, the better prepared you will be to work with the participant.

Data from this interview, and any future assessment information, will need to be securely stored in the participant's file. It is also helpful to include in this file information on the medications the participant is taking (internet search, medication packet insert), their actions but particularly their side effects. It is sensible to be aware of the potential of unintended impact of medication.

All information collected on the participant remains confidential within the ethical and legal guidelines of the practitioner's guiding professional code of ethics. The term confidentiality refers to the principle that the information entrusted to the practitioner must not be disclosed to a third party without the participant or guardian's consent or a clear legal reason. Observing confidentiality is a critical boundary to be respected.

Wellbeing

Wellbeing is the state of being happy. When conducting an assessment of participant wellbeing the practitioner therefore is interested in finding out how the participant feels. Making an accurate assessment of a participant with profound multiple disabilities, including profound motor problems, intellectual and communication impairment, is very difficult. The participant might only be able to communicate: 'via facial expressions, sounds, movements, body posture or muscle tension' (Vos *et al.* 2010, p. 2010) so for the practitioner to accurately determine how the participant is feeling is an unremitting challenge that requires continual validation. It may take a considerable length of time before a practitioner is able to make an accurate assessment. For example smiling might not be an expression of happiness and wellbeing. Some people with disabilities have been conditioned to smile as a social response so they smile whenever they meet someone. The facial expression of smiling might therefore have little connection with the participant's emotions.

A good way to start the wellbeing assessment therefore is to enlist the help of all the participant's key stakeholders and the best time to enlist this support is during the initial interview. The wellbeing questionnaire (see Table 8.2) is specifically designed for the participant stakeholders to complete. However it can also be adapted to help the practitioner's own assessment of participant wellbeing. The questionnaire prompts you to think about the way the participant is behaving and to consider whether this tells you anything about how the participant is feeling.

After the initial interview the practitioner begins the preliminary activity with the participant, and every subsequent activity for that matter, by assessing the participant's wellbeing. The assessment of participant wellbeing then becomes an ongoing focus throughout all practitioner–participant interaction (see Chapter 7). The first time you try to assess the participant's wellbeing you will most probably find yourself completing it in a tentative way. If possible try to make observations and then check them with those made by the key stakeholders. Over time, as you get to know the participant better, you will become faster and more confident at conducting the participant wellbeing assessment and being able to pick up changes during practitioner–participant interactions.

In the unified approach to using multisensory stimulation having an accurate understanding of the participant's wellbeing is essential because wellbeing is a precursor to sense-learning development. When we are content we are more open to new sensory experiences so positive wellbeing facilitates the process. In Chapter 3 we learnt that sensory processing is more complicated than just the processing of sensory information. There is an affective component as well. The way a person feels strongly influences their sensory engagement.

According to Vos *et al.* (2010, p. 1630), people with profound multiple disabilities are 'greatly at risk . . . [of experiencing] low subjective well-being', sensory deprivation and stereotypy.

Table 8.2 Wellbeing questionnaire template

(Modify items on this template to suit your information needs)

Name of participant: _____

Person conducting the interview: _____

Date interview completed: _____

Name(s) of people being interviewed: _____

Relationship to participant (state name): _____

Contact details: _____

Answer the following questions based on your observations of the participant:

Describe how the participant (insert name) has been in general over the past two days.

_____

_____

Have there been times when the participant (insert name) seemed to be happy? If so, when? What indicated the participant was happy? How long did it last?

_____

_____

Did the participant (insert name) smile or laugh? If so, describe:

_____

_____

Have there been times when the participant (insert name) seemed to be unhappy? (If so, when? What indicated the participant was unhappy? How long did it last?

_____

_____

Did the participant (insert name) frown or cry? If so, describe the situation:

_____

_____

Has the participant (insert name) been interested in objects, people, and events? (If so, provide details)

_____

_____

Continued

Continued

Has the participant (insert name) tried to avoid contact with objects, people, and events? (If so, provide details)

_____

_____

Has the participant (insert name) tried to gain the attention of another person? If so, when and how?

_____

_____

What have you been able to tell about the participant (insert name) from his or her facial expressions?

_____

_____

What have you been able to tell about the participant (insert name) from the sounds he or she has made?

_____

_____

What have you been able to tell about the participant (insert name) from his or her body movements or gestures?

_____

_____

What have you been able to tell about the participant (insert name) from his or her posture/muscle tension?

_____

_____

Are there particular issues that could be impacting on participant wellbeing at the moment?

Eating	_____
Constipation	_____
Breathing	_____
Illness	_____
Other	_____

Any other comments you would like to make?

_____

_____

Signature: _____

Stereotypy

Stereotypy is any persistent, highly repetitive or ritualistic behaviour, movement, action or posture. The behaviour seems bizarre, irrelevant and meaningless to observers. Stereotypy is thought to provide predictable gratifying sensorimotor feedback to the individual exhibiting it – although given the sensory fatigue associated with repetition (see Chapter 2) the amount of feedback detected might be quite minimal, or more at a subconscious level.

Stereotypy also occurs in captive animals. It has been associated with home-ostasis (Garner 2005; Hines *et al.* 2008). Homeostasis refers to the body's ability to maintain a stable internal environment in response to environmental changes. It allows an organism to function in a broad range of environmental conditions. When sensory deprivation happens as a result of a combination of severe sense impairment and lack of environmental opportunity, stereotypies emerge, especially when developmental stages have been missed.

Stereotypy is much more prevalent in people with sense-learning disabilities than it is in the general population. In research conducted by Poppes *et al.* (2010), for example, the authors found that 82 per cent of their sample of 181 participants demonstrated stereotypical behaviour. My experience would support this observation. Given this high prevalence, I strongly recommend the practitioner conduct a comprehensive assessment of stereotypy as soon as possible, and keep the situation under review.

As with the assessment of wellbeing, it is best to enlist the support of the key stakeholders. The process of assessment of stereotypies itself provides both the practitioner and the stakeholders with an invaluable opportunity to systematically consider the participant's behaviour from a range of different perspectives. This is particularly important because it encourages the practitioner to work with the stakeholders. Some behaviours are not immediately recognisable as stereo-typies. It can take considerable expertise to recognise them.

An example that might help to illustrate my point is my experience with Lukas. Early in my teaching career I taught a ten-year-old boy who would vomit, at least once a day, for the six months he was in my class. At first it caught me completely by surprise, because nobody had warned me that it would happen. At the time I could not understand why he was vomiting. The behaviour seemed so weird, so unexpected. I did not think it was intentional on Lukas' part so I wondered whether he was ill. I therefore asked his parents to take him for a medical check-up but they told me Lukas had been given a clean bill of health. It was only then that the parents let on that he was vomiting on a regular basis at home as well and they also did not know what to do about it.

It was many years later when researching literature on stereotypy that I appreciated that vomiting could be a stereotypical behaviour. I immediately thought of Lukas. On further reflection I realised Lukas displayed a number of other unusual behaviours that could also fit into the stereotypy description. He would make odd repetitive noises and he would move other students' belongings to the strangest locations. We were forever trying to find where he had put them. At first I thought Lukas was stealing the objects but after a while I realised he was not interested in them at all. He would just move them from one location to another.

My researches on stereotypy have led me to developing the checklist provided (see Table 8.3). This checklist includes a large number of possible stereotypies for you and the key stakeholders to consider. It is presented in tick box format for you to clarify your thinking about stereotypy and to make judgements.

This process starts with the terminology. There has been a long history of these terms being imprecisely defined and so their meanings have tended to be user-dependent. Some of the terms have been used to describe stereotypy are: self-stimulation (sometimes called 'stimming'), self-active engagement, mannerisms, ritualistic behaviour, problem behaviour, challenging behaviour, self-injurious behaviour, blindisms, maladaptive behaviour and obsessive behaviour. To cut through this, I divide stereotypy into three broad categories: self-stimulation, problem behaviours and challenging behaviours.

Self-stimulation refers to persistent, highly repetitive mannerisms unlikely to have any adverse sequelae (i.e. negative pathology). For example John may gently tap his finger on his wrist while he is waiting for the bus each morning, while Julie doodles. The only difference is John has vision impairment and has worked out a different way of fidgeting. Rocking could also be described as self-stimulation. Self-stimulation is not necessarily undesirable as it can help maintain alertness.

Problem behaviours interfere with development and learning. The mannerism becomes so all-consuming that the individual is cut off from the external world. Rocking only becomes problematic when the individual is obsessive, going to extreme lengths to do the behaviour, to the exclusion of other behaviours and he or she finds it almost impossible to stop. The practitioner must therefore assess problem behaviours before the participant goes into the multisensory environment and the practitioner also needs to have a clear plan to manage such behaviour if it starts while the participant is in the space.

Challenging behaviours result in injury to self, to others or to property. Behaviours that may result in community exclusion are also included. Self-injurious behaviour is defined as 'any self-inflicted action that results in bruising, lacerations, lesions, calluses, skin breakdown, or other injury on the individual's own body' (Turner *et al.* 1996, p. 312). It is the intensity, frequency and duration of these behaviours that make them more or less severe. For example rocking would only be thought of as challenging if some damage or injury was occurring or if it was used as a reason to exclude the person from participating in community activities.

In the assessment of stereotypy template (see Table 8.3) the assessor is asked to analyse the participant's behaviour in terms of: intensity, frequency, duration and consequence. Making such judgements is highly subjective so my advice is to work out what interpretation of these terms best suits your purpose. As a

Table 8.3 Assessment of stereotypy template

(Modify items on this template to suit your information needs)

Name of participant: _____

Person conducting the interview: _____

Date interview completed: _____

Name(s) of people being interviewed: _____

Relationship to participant (state name): _____

Contact details: _____

Answer the following questions based on your observations of the participant:
Does the participant currently perform any of the following behaviours?
If so, analyse the behaviour according to whether it is self-stimulation, a
problem or challenging: _____
_____
_____

SS   Self-stimulation, behaviour does not produce any adverse sequelae
PB   Problem behaviour, actions that interfere with development
        and/or learning
CB   Challenging behaviour, actions that result in injury to persons
        and/or property and/or community exclusion
Y/N   Yes/No

Also comment on behaviour in terms of intensity, frequency, duration and
consequence:
I   *Intensity:*
Mi   Mild
Mo   Moderate
Se   Severe
F   *Frequency:*
In   Infrequent (< once a day)
Mf   Moderately frequent (> once a day)
Fr   Frequent (> ten times a day)
D   *Duration:*
Sh   Short periods (< 1 minute)
Mp   Medium periods (1–10 minutes)
Lp   Long periods (> 10 minutes)
O   *Outcome (O):*
Po   Positive
Ze   Zero discernable consequence
Ne   Negative – to self, others, property

Add extra comments if you wish.

Continued

Behaviour	Y/N	SS/PB/CB	Intensity	Frequency	Duration	Outcome	Comments
1 Air swallowing	Y/N	SS/PB/CB	Mi/Mo/Se	In/Mf/Fr	Sh/Mp/Lp	Po/Ze/Ne	
2 Anal/oral behaviour in public	Y/N	SS/PB/CB	Mi/Mo/Se	In/Mf/Fr	Sh/Mp/Lp	Po/Ze/Ne	
3 Bends, bites, grabs, hits, kicks, pinches, punches, slaps, throws, twists object	Y/N	SS/PB/CB	Mi/Mo/Se	In/Mf/Fr	Sh/Mp/Lp	Po/Ze/Ne	
4 Bites, grabs, hits, kicks, pinches, punches, pushes, scratches, slaps others	Y/N	SS/PB/CB	Mi/Mo/Se	In/Mf/Fr	Sh/Mp/Lp	Po/Ze/Ne	
5 Bites, grabs, hits, pinches, punches, slaps self	Y/N	SS/PB/CB	Mi/Mo/Se	In/Mf/Fr	Sh/Mp/Lp	Po/Ze/Ne	
6 Body to object banging	Y/N	SS/PB/CB	Mi/Mo/Se	In/Mf/Fr	Sh/Mp/Lp	Po/Ze/Ne	
7 Bouncing on feet or seat	Y/N	SS/PB/CB	Mi/Mo/Se	In/Mf/Fr	Sh/Mp/Lp	Po/Ze/Ne	
8 Breathing pattern that is radically altered	Y/N	SS/PB/CB	Mi/Mo/Se	In/Mf/Fr	Sh/Mp/Lp	Po/Ze/Ne	
9 Chokes others	Y/N	SS/PB/CB	Mi/Mo/Se	In/Mf/Fr	Sh/Mp/Lp	Po/Ze/Ne	
10 Chokes self	Y/N	SS/PB/CB	Mi/Mo/Se	In/Mf/Fr	Sh/Mp/Lp	Po/Ze/Ne	
11 Clothing manipulated	Y/N	SS/PB/CB	Mi/Mo/Se	In/Mf/Fr	Sh/Mp/Lp	Po/Ze/Ne	
12 Collects and hides things	Y/N	SS/PB/CB	Mi/Mo/Se	In/Mf/Fr	Sh/Mp/Lp	Po/Ze/Ne	
13 Contortions of body parts involving tight sustained flexions	Y/N	SS/PB/CB	Mi/Mo/Se	In/Mf/Fr	Sh/Mp/Lp	Po/Ze/Ne	
14 Cutting self with tools	Y/N	SS/PB/CB	Mi/Mo/Se	In/Mf/Fr	Sh/Mp/Lp	Po/Ze/Ne	
15 Drinking to extreme	Y/N	SS/PB/CB	Mi/Mo/Se	In/Mf/Fr	Sh/Mp/Lp	Po/Ze/Ne	

16 Ear pulling, gouging, pressing on with hands, twisting	Y/N	SS/PB/CB	Mi/Mo/Se	In/Mf/Fr	Sh/Mp/Lp	Po/Ze/Ne
17 Eye crossing	Y/N	SS/PB/CB	Mi/Mo/Se	In/Mf/Fr	Sh/Mp/Lp	Po/Ze/Ne
18 Eye gazing or staring (fixed glassy eye look)	Y/N	SS/PB/CB	Mi/Mo/Se	In/Mf/Fr	Sh/Mp/Lp	Po/Ze/Ne
19 Eye poking, gouging, pressing with hand	Y/N	SS/PB/CB	Mi/Mo/Se	In/Mf/Fr	Sh/Mp/Lp	Po/Ze/Ne
20 Eye rubbing, patting, scratching	Y/N	SS/PB/CB	Mi/Mo/Se	In/Mf/Fr	Sh/Mp/Lp	Po/Ze/Ne
21 Feet tapping on floor, wall, object	Y/N	SS/PB/CB	Mi/Mo/Se	In/Mf/Fr	Sh/Mp/Lp	Po/Ze/Ne
22 Fingers flicked in front of eyes	Y/N	SS/PB/CB	Mi/Mo/Se	In/Mf/Fr	Sh/Mp/Lp	Po/Ze/Ne
23 Finger flicks (not related to eyes)	Y/N	SS/PB/CB	Mi/Mo/Se	In/Mf/Fr	Sh/Mp/Lp	Po/Ze/Ne
24 Grimace – corners of mouth drawn down to reveal upper teeth	Y/N	SS/PB/CB	Mi/Mo/Se	In/Mf/Fr	Sh/Mp/Lp	Po/Ze/Ne
25 Hair pulling	Y/N	SS/PB/CB	Mi/Mo/Se	In/Mf/Fr	Sh/Mp/Lp	Po/Ze/Ne
26 Hair removal	Y/N	SS/PB/CB	Mi/Mo/Se	In/Mf/Fr	Sh/Mp/Lp	Po/Ze/Ne
27 Hand vigorously rubs mouth, face, nose, ears, hair, clothes or objects	Y/N	SS/PB/CB	Mi/Mo/Se	In/Mf/Fr	Sh/Mp/Lp	Po/Ze/Ne
28 Hand wringing – rubbing and clutching each other	Y/N	SS/PB/CB	Mi/Mo/Se	In/Mf/Fr	Sh/Mp/Lp	Po/Ze/Ne
29 Hands locked behind head	Y/N	SS/PB/CB	Mi/Mo/Se	In/Mf/Fr	Sh/Mp/Lp	Po/Ze/Ne
30 Hands moved with continuous flexion and extension	Y/N	SS/PB/CB	Mi/Mo/Se	In/Mf/Fr	Sh/Mp/Lp	Po/Ze/Ne

Continued

© 2012, *The Multisensory Handbook*. Paul Pagliano, Routledge

Continued

Behaviour	Y/N	SS/PB/CB	Intensity	Frequency	Duration	Outcome	Comments
31 Hands waving vertically or horizontally with fingers outstretched in front of eyes	Y/N	SS/PB/CB	Mi/Mo/Se	In/Mf/Fr	Sh/Mp/Lp	Po/Ze/Ne	
32 Head punching/slapping	Y/N	SS/PB/CB	Mi/Mo/Se	In/Mf/Fr	Sh/Mp/Lp	Po/Ze/Ne	
33 Knocking body parts together – ankles, knees, legs, wrists, hands, arms	Y/N	SS/PB/CB	Mi/Mo/Se	In/Mf/Fr	Sh/Mp/Lp	Po/Ze/Ne	
34 Lip chewing	Y/N	SS/PB/CB	Mi/Mo/Se	In/Mf/Fr	Sh/Mp/Lp	Po/Ze/Ne	
35 Makes repetitive non-speech sounds	Y/N	SS/PB/CB	Mi/Mo/Se	In/Mf/Fr	Sh/Mp/Lp	Po/Ze/Ne	
36 Manipulates objects in a ritualistic way – spins, twirls	Y/N	SS/PB/CB	Mi/Mo/Se	In/Mf/Fr	Sh/Mp/Lp	Po/Ze/Ne	
37 Masturbates in public	Y/N	SS/PB/CB	Mi/Mo/Se	In/Mf/Fr	Sh/Mp/Lp	Po/Ze/Ne	
38 Mouthing of objects (holding non-edible objects in contact with the mouth)	Y/N	SS/PB/CB	Mi/Mo/Se	In/Mf/Fr	Sh/Mp/Lp	Po/Ze/Ne	
39 Nail removing	Y/N	SS/PB/CB	Mi/Mo/Se	In/Mf/Fr	Sh/Mp/Lp	Po/Ze/Ne	
40 Pica – placing inedible item (cloth, paper) into the mouth	Y/N	SS/PB/CB	Mi/Mo/Se	In/Mf/Fr	Sh/Mp/Lp	Po/Ze/Ne	
41 Picks up scraps, threads, hair from floor, other surfaces, off other people	Y/N	SS/PB/CB	Mi/Mo/Se	In/Mf/Fr	Sh/Mp/Lp	Po/Ze/Ne	
42 Puts fingers in cavities	Y/N	SS/PB/CB	Mi/Mo/Se	In/Mf/Fr	Sh/Mp/Lp	Po/Ze/Ne	

43 Puts objects in cavities	Y/N	SS/PB/CB	Mi/Mo/Se	In/Mf/Fr	Sh/Mp/Lp	Po/Ze/Ne
44 Rearranges furniture or objects	Y/N	SS/PB/CB	Mi/Mo/Se	In/Mf/Fr	Sh/Mp/Lp	Po/Ze/Ne
45 Rhythmic manipulation of objects by rubbing, rotating, tapping with fingers or body part	Y/N	SS/PB/CB	Mi/Mo/Se	In/Mf/Fr	Sh/Mp/Lp	Po/Ze/Ne
46 Ritualistic head, arm movements	Y/N	SS/PB/CB	Mi/Mo/Se	In/Mf/Fr	Sh/Mp/Lp	Po/Ze/Ne
47 Rocking	Y/N	SS/PB/CB	Mi/Mo/Se	In/Mf/Fr	Sh/Mp/Lp	Po/Ze/Ne
48 Rumination – constantly chewing	Y/N	SS/PB/CB	Mi/Mo/Se	In/Mf/Fr	Sh/Mp/Lp	Po/Ze/Ne
49 Saliva swishing audibly in mouth	Y/N	SS/PB/CB	Mi/Mo/Se	In/Mf/Fr	Sh/Mp/Lp	Po/Ze/Ne
50 Screams not obviously related to distress	Y/N	SS/PB/CB	Mi/Mo/Se	In/Mf/Fr	Sh/Mp/Lp	Po/Ze/Ne
51 Skin picking	Y/N	SS/PB/CB	Mi/Mo/Se	In/Mf/Fr	Sh/Mp/Lp	Po/Ze/Ne
52 Spins on equipment (chair)	Y/N	SS/PB/CB	Mi/Mo/Se	In/Mf/Fr	Sh/Mp/Lp	Po/Ze/Ne
53 Spins while standing	Y/N	SS/PB/CB	Mi/Mo/Se	In/Mf/Fr	Sh/Mp/Lp	Po/Ze/Ne
54 Spits at others	Y/N	SS/PB/CB	Mi/Mo/Se	In/Mf/Fr	Sh/Mp/Lp	Po/Ze/Ne
55 Sways head	Y/N	SS/PB/CB	Mi/Mo/Se	In/Mf/Fr	Sh/Mp/Lp	Po/Ze/Ne
56 Sways torso	Y/N	SS/PB/CB	Mi/Mo/Se	In/Mf/Fr	Sh/Mp/Lp	Po/Ze/Ne
57 Teeth banging	Y/N	SS/PB/CB	Mi/Mo/Se	In/Mf/Fr	Sh/Mp/Lp	Po/Ze/Ne
58 Teeth clicking – audibly and rapidly closing teeth together	Y/N	SS/PB/CB	Mi/Mo/Se	In/Mf/Fr	Sh/Mp/Lp	Po/Ze/Ne
59 Teeth grinding	Y/N	SS/PB/CB	Mi/Mo/Se	In/Mf/Fr	Sh/Mp/Lp	Po/Ze/Ne
60 Throws objects at people	Y/N	SS/PB/CB	Mi/Mo/Se	In/Mf/Fr	Sh/Mp/Lp	Po/Ze/Ne

Continued

Continued

Behaviour	Y/N	SS/PB/CB	Intensity	Frequency	Duration	Outcome	Comments
61 Tongue rolling and clicking	Y/N	SS/PB/CB	Mi/Mo/Se	In/Mf/Fr	Sh/Mp/Lp	Po/Ze/Ne	
62 Touches others in inappropriate ways	Y/N	SS/PB/CB	Mi/Mo/Se	In/Mf/Fr	Sh/Mp/Lp	Po/Ze/Ne	
63 Touches self, objects, others	Y/N	SS/PB/CB	Mi/Mo/Se	In/Mf/Fr	Sh/Mp/Lp	Po/Ze/Ne	
64 Verbal abuse	Y/N	SS/PB/CB	Mi/Mo/Se	In/Mf/Fr	Sh/Mp/Lp	Po/Ze/Ne	
65 Vomiting	Y/N	SS/PB/CB	Mi/Mo/Se	In/Mf/Fr	Sh/Mp/Lp	Po/Ze/Ne	
Other (please describe)	Y/N	SS/PB/CB	Mi/Mo/Se	In/Mf/Fr	Sh/Mp/Lp	Po/Ze/Ne	
	Y/N	SS/PB/CB	Mi/Mo/Se	In/Mf/Fr	Sh/Mp/Lp	Po/Ze/Ne	
	Y/N	SS/PB/CB	Mi/Mo/Se	In/Mf/Fr	Sh/Mp/Lp	Po/Ze/Ne	
	Y/N	SS/PB/CB	Mi/Mo/Se	In/Mf/Fr	Sh/Mp/Lp	Po/Ze/Ne	

Signature: _____

guideline, however, intensity is thought to be mild if the participant is easily distracted from the behaviour, moderate if it takes several more concerted attempts to distract the participant from doing the behaviour and severe if the practitioner is unable to distract the participant. Frequency is determined to be infrequent if it is less than once a day, moderately frequent if it is once a day or greater and frequent if it is more than ten times a day. Duration is determined to be short periods if it is less than one minute, medium periods if it is between one to ten minutes and long periods if it continues uninterrupted for more than ten minutes.

Lukas' vomiting was moderately frequent because it happened at least once a day (at school, although it seemed to be occurring daily at home as well). The vomiting episode was fairly quick so it only occurred over short periods of time. However I never managed to distract him or prevent the vomiting so it was of a severe intensity. There were a number of negative consequences to the vomiting. He was clearly disgorging his food before it was being fully digested so there was a problem with him receiving adequate nutrition. Also the vomiting made it particularly difficult to take him out in public, so it was a challenging behaviour.

Engagement

Engagement is an operational state of being purposefully psychologically active. This is in direct contrast to the 'down time' described in Chapter 3 where the inhabitants of the village were 'doing nothing', slumped and passive. Engagement is a prerequisite for learning.

Engagement in participants who have few communication skills can only be assessed by careful observation of behaviour. Behaviour is taken to be an action or deed performed by a person. Behaviour can be classified into deeds that non-purposeful and those that are purposeful.

Bunning (1998) describes three types of non-purposeful behaviours as:

1 Body actions where the individual is not conscious. These actions might occur during sleep, deep rest, as a result of sedation or during an epileptic fit.
2 Routine unconscious body movements that happen spontaneously during waking hours, such as yawning or inadvertently scratching one's head.
3 Stereotypies.

Purposeful behaviour comprises actions performed for a deliberate reason. The person doing the behaviour had a conscious intention that led to the behaviour being instigated; there was some form of motivation behind the behaviour being performed. When a person produces a purposeful behaviour, this is indicative of engagement.

The goal when using multisensory stimulation with a participant is to decrease the amount of non-purposeful behaviour and to increase the amount of purposeful behaviour. As discussed earlier in this chapter, three motivations behind purposeful behaviour are: a will to pleasure, a will to power and a will to meaning. Individuals purposefully engage with sensory stimulation, objects, people and events through their senses.

An example of engagement with sensory stimulation is a participant seeing a light and smiling. The participant engages with the stimulation and achieves an in-the-moment pleasure filled experience that produces a true smile. The person then purposefully chooses to continue looking at the light.

An example of object-engagement (purposeful interaction with an object) is the participant playing with a fibre optic spray. The manipulation of the object helps to prolong the in-the-moment pleasure that comes from seeing the light.

An example of person-engagement (purposeful interaction with another person) is interaction with the practitioner. The participant makes eye contact with the practitioner and spontaneously smiles a true smile.

Event-engagement refers to the individual participating in a particular event, such as having a massage. Here the event is defined as an interconnected chain of occurrences.

Object-person-engagement occurs when the purposeful interaction is with both a person and with an object, for example, when two participants are in the ball pool and they pass a ball from one to the other.

Bunning (1996) subdivides engagement into five levels of involvement: orientation, responsiveness, reciprocation, initiative and association. These can be determined in the following ways:

- Orientation: this is passive basic awareness. Has information about an offer to engage been received? Does the participant become activated? Does the participant stop self-stimulation in response to the offer to engage?
- Responsiveness: this is active basic awareness. Does the participant respond to received sense information? Is the response positive, neutral or negative?
- Reciprocation: is there an interchange of interaction, such as turn taking?
- Initiative: is the participant adding new information?
- Association: is the participant making a connection of some kind, for example gratifying behaviour, instrumental behaviour or meaningful behaviour?

The questionnaire on engagement prompts a systematic appraisal of the participant's engagement (see Table 8.4). If the participant is not sufficiently engaged, then this must be addressed before other activities take place.

Assessing the senses

Assessing the senses involves the evaluation of the participant's ability in interoception and exteroception. Two different assessment protocols have been adopted. This is because the majority of sensory processing for interoception happens at an unconscious level and the majority of processing of the senses of

Table 8.4 Engagement template

(Modify items on this template to suit your information needs)

Name of participant: _____

Person conducting the assessment: _____

Date: _____

Answer the following questions based on your observations of the participant:

Level of engagement – with sensory stimulation (SS), object (O), person (P) and event (E)

Level		Type of sensory stimulation	Object	Person	Events	Comments
Orientation						
	Has information about offers to engage been received?					
	Does participant stop self-stimulation in response to offers to engage?					
Responsiveness						
	Does participant respond to sense information on offer?					
	Is the response positive, neutral or negative?					
Reciprocation						
	Is there turn taking?					
Initiative						
	Is the participant adding new information?					
Association						
	Is participant making a connection of some kind – e.g. generalising, aware of object permanence, linking people and events?					

Other comments: _____

Signature: _____

exteroception occurs at a conscious level. The order of assessment activities, starting with interoception, and then moving on to exteroception near and exteroception distant (see Figure 8.2) is consistent with the way development takes place. Whenever possible, the order within each sense area also adheres to the natural developmental stages. This not only provides the practitioner with a template with which to assess the participant, but it also helps to inform the practitioner as to what are the most likely next developmental steps for the participant.

Interoception

Interoception encompasses proprioception, the vestibular sense and any other sense receptor stimulated from within the body. Like all sense activity the senses of interoception provide important stimulation that directly impacts on brain development. They also play a significant role in enhancing quality of life.

The assessment template for interoception merely provides the practitioner with a general overview (see Table 8.5). It is really a check to see if a more comprehensive assessment is required. This would need to be conducted by a physiotherapist, an occupational therapist, an audiologist (for a vestibular assessment) or a medical practitioner. This is because of the specialised nature of the required interventions. It would therefore be very helpful for the practitioner to work with these specialists to plan the best programme for the participant.

The interoception assessment template looks at functions such as breathing, cardiovascular stability, neurological stability, temperature control, thirst and hunger, the mechanics of swallowing, digestion, bladder and bowel function.

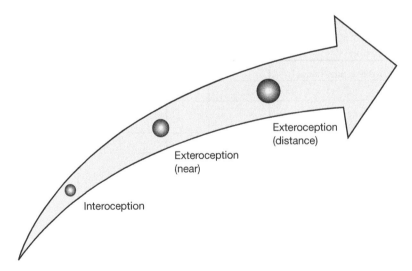

Figure 8.2 The emergence of the senses in the developing organism.

Table 8.5 Interoception template

(Modify items on this template to suit your information needs)

Name of participant: _____
Person conducting the assessment: _____
Date: _____

Answer the following questions based on your observations of the participant:

Check participant records to identify what is already known about the participant's:
Proprioception
Vestibular sense
Other internal sense organs

Physiotherapist's report: ATTACHED/NOT ATTACHED
Occupational therapist's report: ATTACHED/NOT ATTACHED
Speech language pathologist's report: ATTACHED/NOT ATTACHED

Answer the following questions based on your observations of the participant:

Modality	Normal/ abnormal (N/A)	Comments	Specialist intervention required (Y/N)
Breathing			
Cardiovascular stability (e.g. faints)			
Neurological stability (e.g. fits, tics)			
Temperature control			
Thirst			
Hunger			
Swallowing			
Vomiting			
Excessive bloating			
Bladder function			
Bowel function			
Other			

Continued

© 2012, *The Multisensory Handbook*. Paul Pagliano, Routledge

Continued

Current status:

Which describes the participant's current level of motor development?

Extension against gravity
- ❏ Lifting head and straightening trunk in prone position
- ❏ Lifting head and straightening trunk in supine position

Limb movements
- ❏ Flexing/extending R (right) arm/shoulder
- ❏ Flexing/extending L (left) arm/shoulder
- ❏ Flexing/extending R leg/hip
- ❏ Flexing/extending L leg/hip
- ❏ Coordinated bilateral arms together
- ❏ Coordinated bilateral legs together

- ❏ R   Coordinated arm and leg together, same side (circle)
- ❏ L

- ❏ R+L Coordinated arm and leg together, different sides (circle)
- ❏ L+R

Body movement through space
- ❏ Front to back
- ❏ Side to side
- ❏ Rotary

Using support for balancing
- ❏ Lying
- ❏ Sitting
- ❏ Crawling
- ❏ Standing
- ❏ Walking

Which activities are popular with the participant?
- ❏ Ball pool
- ❏ Rocking
- ❏ Spinning
- ❏ Swaying
- ❏ Swimming pool
- ❏ Swinging
- ❏ Water bed
- ❏ Others (list)

What movements will the participant voluntarily engage in?
- ❏ Reach
- ❏ Reach to touch
- ❏ Grasp
- ❏ Reach to grasp
- ❏ Hand (touch)–eye coordination
- ❏ Release
- ❏ Others (list)

What is the best interoceptive environment for the participant?
Checklist
- ❏ Time of day
- ❏ Muscular activity
- ❏ Balance
- ❏ Length of activity

Other comments: _____

_____

_____

_____

Signature: _____

These are all areas that can usually only be significantly improved by specialist intervention, independent of the caring practitioner.

The template also looks at posture and muscle control. Children develop control over their physical bodies in progressions: head to tail, trunk to finger tips/toes, joint flexion to extension, reflexes to purposeful movement. Following this, sensorimotor development follows four further sets of progressions (Bly 1983). These are:

1 Extension against gravity – lifting head and straightening trunk while in prone position then lifting head and bending trunk while in supine position.
2 Increasingly complex combinations of limb movements, random to coordinated bilateral arm and leg movements, to unilateral arm and leg movements, to diagonal arm and leg movements.
3 Body movements through space, front–back, then side to side, then rotary.
4 Large support base for balancing, which progressively diminishes in size as equilibrium is achieved.

Working with a physiotherapist identifies the areas that need attention. The physiotherapist and the occupational therapist will provide the practitioner with strategies to help guide the participant to more actively engage in the controlled multisensory environment.

Exteroception

For assessment purposes the senses of exteroception have been organised into four groups. They are: chemosensation, the tactual and the somatic senses, hearing, and vision. Useful descriptions of these senses can be found in Chapter 2. When assessing the senses of exteroception the initial goal is to identify whether the participant is able to detect the particular sense sensation; if so, is he or she able to recognise it? And if so, is he or she able to differentiate it from other similar sensory experiences? Once the participant is able to differentiate sense information this then leads to the development of basic concepts. A number of the listed basic concepts apply to most or even all the senses of exteroception. These include: same and different, more and less, stop and start, and on and off. Some other basic concepts are much more sense specific. These include: hot and cold (for temperature), and loud and soft (for hearing). The practitioner is also invited to build on these basic concepts (see Tables 8.6–8.10).

The template begins with chemosensation (see Table 8.6). After the initial assessment regarding sense thresholds the practitioner is asked about the participant's ability to suck, chew and swallow. This is followed by questions regarding whether the participant shows any evidence of chemosensation sensitivity, avoidance or defensiveness and to give examples. The practitioner is also asked to list eating and drinking preferences, to catalogue the participant's taste and smell likes and dislikes and to think about ideal environments for the participant. The section on chemosensation concludes with an assessment of functional taste and smell.

The second sense group for detailed assessment is the somatic senses of touch, pressure, temperature and pain (see Table 8.7). These senses are sometimes referred to the tactual and cutaneous senses. This template follows a similar order to the chemosensation template, starting with sensory thresholds and basic concepts. The practitioner is then asked to make links back to proprioceptive development and to consider whether the participant exhibits any features of tactile sensitivity, avoidance or defensiveness. Next the practitioner is asked to focus attention onto each somatic sense before cataloguing the participant's somatic senses likes and dislikes. The section concludes with an assessment of optimum environments and functional touch.

The third sense area is hearing (see Table 8.8). This template begins with assessment of sense thresholds, basic concepts and checking reports from the audiologist (including audiogram), otorhinolaryngologist (ear, nose and throat specialist) and the participant's file. These reports enable the practitioner to clarify the participant's degree of hearing loss. This is followed by questions regarding whether aids for hearing are used such as hearing aids or a cochlear implant. The practitioner is also asked to assess what is the participant's best listening

Table 8.6 Exteroception template – chemosensation

(Modify items on this template to suit your information needs)

Name of participant: _____

Person conducting the assessment: _____

Date: _____

Answer the following questions based on your observations of the participant: Adjust to fit each type of chemosensation being assessed, e.g. taste, smell, chemical:

Sense	Type	Type	Type
No detection			
Detection			
Recognition			
Differentiation			
Basic concepts			
Same/different			
More/less			
Start/stop			
Big/small			
Hot/cold			
Before/after			
Wet/dry			
Smooth/rough			
Soft/hard			
Strong/weak			
Yes/no			
Like/dislike			
Nominate other relevant basic concepts:			

Continued

Continued

Observe and comment on the participant's ability to:

Suck	
Chew	
Swallow	

Is the participant showing evidence of chemosensation sensitivity, avoidance or defensiveness?
If so, give examples.

Eating/drinking preferences:

Favourite food(s)	
Favourite drink(s)	
Which foods does participant refuse to eat	
— Suggestions why?	
Which drinks des participant refuse to drink	
— Suggestions why?	

Update on the participant's taste and smell likes and dislikes:

Tastes				Comments
Sweet (honey)	☺	☺	☹	
Sweet (sugar)	☺	☺	☹	
Salt (anchovies)	☺	☺	☹	
Salt (crisps)	☺	☺	☹	
Sour (lemon juice)	☺	☺	☹	
Sour (grapefruit piece)	☺	☺	☹	
Bitter (angostura bitters)	☺	☺	☹	
Bitter (endive)	☺	☺	☹	
Soft textures (yoghurt)	☺	☺	☹	
Solid textures (apple)	☺	☺	☹	
Cold (ice cream)	☺	☺	☹	

Room temperature (water)	☺	😐	☹
Warm temperature (custard)	☺	😐	☹
Chilli (mild chilli beans)	☺	😐	☹
Menthol	☺	😐	☹
Milk (cold)	☺	😐	☹
Orange juice (room temperature)	☺	😐	☹
Chocolate drink (warm)	☺	😐	☹

Smells				Comments
Basil (arousing)	☺	😐	☹	
Chamomile (relaxing)	☺	😐	☹	
Cinnamon (arousing)	☺	😐	☹	
Clary sage (arousing)	☺	😐	☹	
Eucalyptus (relaxing)	☺	😐	☹	
Frankincense (relaxing)	☺	😐	☹	
Lavender (relaxing)	☺	😐	☹	
Lemon (arousing)	☺	😐	☹	
Patchouli (arousing)	☺	😐	☹	
Peppermint (arousing)	☺	😐	☹	
Rose (relaxing)	☺	😐	☹	
Rosemary (arousing)	☺	😐	☹	
Ylang-ylang (relaxing)	☺	😐	☹	

Other smell and taste experiences				Comments
	☺	😐	☹	
	☺	😐	☹	
	☺	😐	☹	
	☺	😐	☹	

What are the best taste and smell environments for the participant?

Checklist
- ❏ Time of day
- ❏ Taste
- ❏ Smell
- ❏ Length of activity
- ❏ During meal times

Continued

Continued

Functional taste and smell

Taste and smell skill level	Comments
Taste/smell awareness	
Taste/smell attending	
Taste/smell localising	
Taste/smell recognition	
Taste/smell understanding	

Other comments: _____

_____

_____

Signature: _____

Table 8.7 Exteroception template – somatic senses

(Modify items on this template to suit your information needs)

Name of participant: _____

Person conducting the assessment: _____

Date: _____

Answer the following questions based on your observations of the participant: Adjust to fit each type of somatic sense being assessed (touch, temperature, pressure and pain):

Sense	Type	Type	Type
No detection			
Detection			
Recognition			
Differentiation			
Basic concepts			
Same/different			
More/less			

Start/stop			
On/off			
Big/small			
Hot/cold			
High low/up down			
Before/after			
Top/bottom			
Far/near			
Fast/slow			
Wet/dry			
Clean/dirty			
Smooth/rough			
Soft/hard			
Heavy/light			
Strong/weak			
Yes/no			
Like/dislike			
In/out			
Middle (in-between)			
Direction			
Nominate other relevant basic concepts:			

Does participant require more work on functional proprioception?
Is the participant showing evidence of tactile sensitivity, avoidance or defensiveness?
If so, give examples.
Is the participant aware of pressure?
Is the participant aware of changes in temperature? What is the participant's preferred room temperature?
How does participant express that he or she is in pain? How do you know?
What supporting evidence do you have?

Continued

Continued

Update on the participant's somatic senses likes and dislikes

Touch experiences				Comments
Textures (rough to smooth)				
Coarse sandpaper	☺	☹	☹	
Velvet	☺	☹	☹	
Density (hard to soft)				
Glass	☺	☹	☹	
Sponge	☺	☹	☹	
State (gas to fluid to solid)				
Fan	☺	☹	☹	
Milk	☺	☹	☹	
Apple	☺	☹	☹	
Surface to depth (palpation)				
Feel something with gloves on	☺	☹	☹	
Size (small to large)	☺	☹	☹	
Sand	☺	☹	☹	
Rocks	☺	☹	☹	
Temperature (hot to cold)				
Hot water bottle	☺	☹	☹	
Ice	☺	☹	☹	
Vibration (static, gentle, vigorous)				
Vibrator – stopped	☺	☹	☹	
Vibrator – slow	☺	☹	☹	
Vibrator – fast	☺	☹	☹	
Shape (circle, square)				

Other touch experiences				Comments
	☺	☹	☹	
	☺	☹	☹	
	☺	☹	☹	
	☺	☹	☹	

What are the best somatic environments (touch, pressure, temperature, pain) for the participant?

Checklist
- ❏　Time of day
- ❏　Touch
- ❏　Pressure
- ❏　Temperature
- ❏　Pain
- ❏　Length of activity
- ❏　Background interference

Functional touch
Locating – random or intentional search for object
Exploring object
Manipulation of object
Recognition of object tactually
Comparison – showing preference or rejection of objects
Communication – using object to signal
Organising – set place/task for objects

Other comments: _____
_____
_____
_____

Signature: _____

environment and whether there is any evidence of hearing sensitivity, avoidance or defensiveness. The section concludes with information on the participant's auditory skill level.

The fourth sense area for more detailed assessment is vision (see Table 8.9). Like hearing this begins with assessment of thresholds and basic concepts, and checking on reports from the optometrist, the ophthalmologist and the participant's file. These reports provide the practitioner with details regarding the participant's type of vision loss. This is followed by information about whether visual aids have been prescribed and are being used. The practitioner is also asked to assess what is the participant's best visual environment and whether there is any evidence of vision sensitivity, avoidance or defensiveness. The assessment concludes with information on the participant's visual skill level.

Table 8.8 Exteroception template – hearing

(Modify items on this template to suit your information needs)

Name of participant: _____

Person conducting the assessment: _____

Date: _____

Answer the following questions based on your observations of the participant:
Adjust to fit each sub-type of hearing being assessed:

Sense	Sub-type	Sub-type	Sub-type
No detection			
Detection			
Recognition			
Differentiation			
Basic concepts			
Same/different			
More/less			
Start/stop			
On/off			
Big/small			
High low/up down			
Loud/soft			
Before/after			
Top/bottom			
Far/near			
Fast/slow			
Soft/hard			
Yes/no			
Like/dislike			
In/out			
Middle (in-between)			
Direction			

Nominate other relevant basic concepts:			

Functional hearing

Audiologist's report (plus audiogram):   ATTACHED/NOT ATTACHED
Otorhinolaryngologist's report: ATTACHED/NOT ATTACHED
Participant's file (hearing issues):   ATTACHED/NOT ATTACHED

Degree of hearing loss	Educationally deaf (no functional hearing)
	Hard of hearing
	Limited hearing

Type of hearing loss	Conductive loss
	Sensorineural hearing loss
	Mixed hearing loss
	Central/cortical hearing loss

What aids have been prescribed to help hearing? Is the participant wearing/using them?

Does participant have a cochlear implant?

What is the best listening environment for the participant?

Checklist
❏   Time of day
❏   Volume
❏   Pitch
❏   Length of listening
❏   Background noise

Is the participant showing evidence of auditory sensitivity, avoidance or defensiveness?

If so, give examples.

Continued

Continued

What auditory skill level has the participant reached?

Auditory skill level	Comments
Auditory awareness	
Auditory attending	
Auditory localising	
Auditory recognition	
Auditory understanding	

Other comments: _____

_____

_____

_____

Signature: _____

Table 8.9 Exteroception template – vision

(Modify items on this template to suit your information needs)

Name of participant: _____

Person conducting the assessment: _____

Date: _____

Answer the following questions based on your observations of the participant: Adjust to fit each sub-type of vision being assessed:

Sense	Sub-type	Sub-type	Sub-type
No detection			
Detection			
Recognition			
Differentiation			
Basic concepts			
Same/different			

More/less			
Start/stop			
On/off			
Big/small			
High low/up down			
Loud/soft			
Before/after			
Top/bottom			
Far/near			
Fast/slow			
Clean/dirty			
Smooth/rough			
Heavy/light			
Strong/weak			
Yes/no			
Like/dislike			
In/out			
Middle (in-between)			
Direction			
Nominate other relevant basic concepts:			

Functional vision
Optometrist's report: ATTACHED/NOT ATTACHED
Ophthalmologist's report: ATTACHED/NOT ATTACHED
Participant's file (vision issues):   ATTACHED/NOT ATTACHED

Continued

Continued

Degree of vision loss	Educationally blind (no functional vision)
	Low vision
	Visually limited
Type of vision loss	Field of vision
	Distance visual acuity
	Near visual acuity
	Stereopsis
	Colour vision
	Accommodation/fusional vergence
	Ocular motility: saccades, tracking
	Near point of convergence
	Cortical visual impairment

What aids have been prescribed to help vision, e.g. glasses, contact lens, low vision aids? Is the participant wearing/using them?

Prescription:

What is the best visual environment for the participant?

Checklist
- ❏ Time of day
- ❏ Image size and intensity
- ❏ Image location and complexity
- ❏ Colours
- ❏ Lighting
- ❏ Background stimuli
- ❏ Movement
- ❏ Length of viewing

Is the participant showing evidence of visual sensitivity, avoidance or defensiveness?

If so, give examples.

'Sensory potential' means that the sense organ has some function, even though it may well be severely impaired. It is clearly highly desirable that this function be made as optimum as it can be through ongoing therapist/medical intervention providing specific aids, surgery and/or medications as appropriate (see Chapter 8). Sensory potential is a prerequisite for sensory detection.

So if a participant is thought to have sensory potential, but he or she does not demonstrate evidence of positive engagement (see Chapter 8), then the practitioner designs stimulation to specifically promote development of that sense. The practitioner is aiming to build up the participant's pool of relevant pleasurable sensory experiences (see Chapter 3) to induce a tipping point (see Chapter 5). The desired tipping point is a transition in sensory processing to detection, a new way of experiencing the world.

After activating the sense organ, sensory stimulation travels along pathway connections (see Chapter 4) from the sense organ to the brain and within the brain. For detection to occur there must be the initial learning 'of' the sense (the establishment and laying down of these sensory pathway connections). For the sense experience to be detected, the practitioner therefore redesigns the environment to achieve three outcomes. These are: to establish pathway connections from the sense organ to the brain, for it to be pleasurable and to induce a tipping point.

The practitioner starts to achieve these three outcomes through the use of Mere Exposure Theory, in this context the idea that the more familiarity a person has with a sensory stimulus the more likely it is that person will grow to like the stimulus. Furthermore if this exposure occurs within the remit of a caring professional and in a trusted environment, then the benefit is likely to be even more pronounced.

Robert Zajonc's historic research on the concept's significance using chickens is particularly enlightening and illustrative (Zajonc 1968). It involved playing one of two different musical tones to two sets of fertile eggs. Upon hatching, the chickens reliably chose the tone played to them when they were hatching in preference to the tone they had not previously heard. The exciting research implication is that mere exposure is effective even if there is little, if any, cognition.

People have long known that being in the presence of the familiar can be enormously comforting, especially for young children. A famous example of this is a comfort object such as a much-loved soft toy, which is used to help the infant make a transition from the safety and security of a known environment with known people to the relative uncertainty of a new environment with unknown people, such as starting kindergarten (Dell'Orto 2003). Winnicott (1971) argues that the comfort object takes on some of the characteristics of the caring bond between the mother and child. I argue that the comfort object is a tool for the caring practitioner but no substitute.

The caring practitioner uses this biological predilection for being attracted to the familiar to present simple non-threatening pleasurable stimulation repeatedly in a controlled sensory environment. This stimulation is designed to appeal to the sensory potential of the participant. The effect of that stimulation is carefully monitored and initially adjusted if necessary. However a precision of similarity in the repetitions is vital to establish and strengthen sensory pathway connections.

I now want to describe a particular case where redesign was put into action. At the time of the redesign intervention, José was two years old. He was born able to hear but, following a traumatic accident that left him in a coma for four weeks, he was no longer noticeably responding to sounds.

Hilary, his therapist, decided to use Mere Exposure Theory as a way to try to trigger auditory development. She chose a large Tibetan singing bowl. Hilary reasoned the low beautiful harmonics produced by the bowl would make it easier for José to eventually detect the sounds. Also she herself loved the sounds it made so she felt she would be able to persevere with striking the bowl the large number of times she anticipated would be necessary to start getting José to listen.

Each morning when José arrived for therapy, Hilary would begin the day's activities by laying him on a resonance board (Nielsen 1992). A resonance board is made of plywood and specifically designed to give a participant with sensory disabilities greatly enhanced auditory feedback (see Brown 2002/2003) for instructions on how to construct a resonance board). Once José was comfortable on the resonance board Hilary would place the singing bowl just beside the top of his head.

Hilary would then strike the bowl and allow it to fully reverberate for a total of twenty-one times. José never objected so she continued the activity for six weeks until one day when she struck the bowl he slightly moved his head in Hilary's direction. Hilary took this to mean that José was beginning to consciously detect the sound. She was therefore delighted to observe the same movement become more deliberate and pronounced over the following two weeks.

As Hilary continued the activity she noticed that José seemed to enjoy the sound the singing bowl made more and more. His hand tremor would gradually subside while she played the bowl. Unfortunately it would return a few minutes after she finished but still she felt she now had enough evidence to reassure her that she was on the right track. She therefore reasoned it was time to introduce a new sound for José to detect and recognise, a completely different sound. This time she chose a large tambourine hand drum, which she would hold just above José's chest and beat a further twenty-one times. She always started the day with the singing bowl and then moved on to the tambourine. This time José was considerably faster at showing evidence that he detected the sound and soon he was also demonstrating evidence that he could recognise the two sets of sounds.

Function-centred design

With function-centred design the caring practitioner's focus is on promoting more effective participant functioning. For example the practitioner might be interested in helping the participant overcome debilitating problems associated with sensory sensitivity and sensory defensiveness.

Once again Mere Exposure Theory can be employed. An important research finding of Mere Exposure Theory is that over time Mere Exposure can be used to change a person's feeling towards a certain stimulus from dislike to like (Zajonc 2001). This process is similar to how a person develops an acquired taste. It also helps to explain how people from one culture come to love foods that neighbouring cultures regard as stomach-churning, a celebrated example being *surströmming*, an extremely strong smelling distinctively flavoured fermented Baltic herring that is much prized in Sweden.

In the multisensory environment the caring practitioner uses Mere Exposure Theory in conjunction with graduated exposure therapy or systematic desensitisation (Wolpe 1958). This involves the caring practitioner coupling a nearby pleasant stimulus with a distant negative stimulus and very gradually, over an extended period of time, bringing the negative stimulus closer to the participant while retaining the positive stimulus nearby (Jones 1924).

South (2001) describes how she successfully used graduated exposure over twenty-four sessions with a four-year-old boy with autism with tactile defensiveness to get him to better tolerate a skin care product. Sessions began, ended and were interspersed with highly regarded games. The gradual introduction began by just locating a bottle of lotion on a distant table. A discussion about its funny shape was followed by a game and bringing the bottle a little closer. When the bottle became part of the game it was brought even closer. Eventually the child willingly applied the lotion onto his own hands and rubbed it in.

Simplicity whenever possible

The simplicity whenever possible design strategy was introduced to ensure that the multisensory environment never becomes too complicated. The caring practitioner must be able to control the environment in ways that are relevant for the participant and if the environment is too complicated the practitioner will find it difficult to be able to spontaneously and appropriately respond to participant needs.

The assessment templates (see Tables 8.1 to 8.9) were developed with the simplicity whenever possible strategy in mind. For example in Table 8.6 the practitioner is asked to keep a simple record of participant taste and smell experiences. The template helps to provide the practitioner with a simple guideline to follow regarding how to help expand the participant's repertoire of taste and smell experiences. The template also makes it easier to track changes over time.

Multiple methods to achieve the same outcome

The idea behind the multiple methods to achieve the same outcome design approach is if one strategy set does not work then another set might. This approach is based on the mastery learning assumption, which is that all participants can learn providing the right environmental conditions are provided (Gusky and Gates 1986). It is therefore the caring practitioner's job to try to design an environment with the right learning conditions for a particular participant. Here the focus is on participant achievement.

In Chapter 6 I used the example of Chaos Theory and Complexity Theory to illustrate how I worked with a bee to help it escape a room. Now I would like to describe another strategy set that could be used with the participant to promote mastery learning, that of the nine stages of skill development (Kozloff and Rice 1998). These nine stages are:

1   Pre-acquisition: with pre-acquisition the participant demonstrates learning potential and readiness but the skill has not yet been acquired. The practitioner assesses learning potential and readiness by carefully considering what ability is required for the participant to acquire the skill. For example the goal might be for the participant to detect a bright light made by a flashlight in the dark room. The practitioner would therefore need to find out from an ophthalmologist and an optometrist about the participant's potential for vision in these circumstances.

2   Acquisition: this is where the participant learns the basic components of a skill. If the skill to be taught is for the participant to be able to detect a bright light made by a flashlight (torch) in the dark room then the basic components of the skill would involve being able to accurately detect if the light was on or if the light was off.

3   Fluency: this is where the participant learns to perform the skill accurately and proficiently. With repetition the participant might become better at being able to tell if the flashlight is on or off and may even to be able to determine when it comes on and when it goes off.

4   Endurance: this is where the practitioner thinks about the duration of the activity, whether the participant is able to engage in the skill for an extended period of time. Learning a new skill can be tiring so it takes multiple repetitions before the participant builds up sufficient stamina to be able to engage in the skill for longer time periods.

5   Momentum: up to this point the learning has been designed in its purest form. There have been no distractions – just the dark room and the flashlight turning on and off. Once the participant has reached this stage of skill development the practitioner is able to introduce a distraction to ascertain whether the participant is still able to continue to engage in the activity. This is a critical stage of skill development because below this level any other sensory stimulation would disrupt the skill development. During stages one to four the practitioner is strongly advised not to speak to the participant or to change the stimulation in any way.

6   Generalisation: this is when the participant is able to transfer the skill learnt in one environment to another environment. For example the participant

may now be able to detect the same flashlight that was originally detected in the dark room at night at home.

7   Adaptation: this is where the participant is able to modify the skill in some way to make it more personally relevant and meaningful. For example the participant might be able to cover the face of the flashlight when it is switched on so it can no longer be detected and then uncover it so that it can be detected. The ability to play with the skill is a significant time when the participant starts to demonstrate ownership of the learning.

8   Retention: this is where the participant retains all seven previously learnt aspects of the skill over an extended period of time. Now the practitioner might only show the flashlight to the participant in the dark room occasionally just to check whether the participant can still detect the light.

9   Maintenance: the participant has now achieved independence and does not need the practitioner's assistance.

Slow design

The central focus of slow design is to create an environment that enhances participant wellbeing (see Chapter 3). This wellbeing is seen as a prerequisite for learning and development. For learning and development to take place the participant must be able to achieve success in some form. This is critical to the use of slow design because the intention of slow design is to promote intrinsic motivation. Motivation is the incentive that induces a person to act. Extrinsic motivation is any driving force that comes from outside the individual such as encouragement from others. Intrinsic motivation is the driving force that comes from within the individual so it is associated with the pleasure that comes from successfully doing the activity.

Seligman (1975) describes learned helplessness as the situation where repeated failure causes an individual to identify with the failure and to cease to initiate any further interaction. Learned helplessness, Seligman (1998) argues, can be overcome by providing the participant with an abundance of success experiences. An abundance of success helps to lead the participant to a state of absorption, what Mihaly Csikszentmihalyi (1990) describes as flow. Flow is achieved when the participant's best skill level matches the task difficulty. Low skill level and low challenge result in participant apathy. Increasing the skill level while retaining a low challenge for the participant takes the participant into boredom and then into relaxation. Alternatively increasing challenge while retaining low skill level takes the participant into worry and then into anxiety. When both skill level and challenge are increased simultaneously the participant moves from apathy through arousal and control into flow. This model therefore provides the practitioner with a clear set of guidelines to follow when using the multisensory environment.

With flow the important point to remember is skill level and challenge are both relative to the participant. For a participant who has only just passed through the sense detection threshold, the practitioner would therefore need to go back to the nine stages of skill development to work out how best to increase the challenge and maintain flow, for example to develop fluency, endurance, momentum, generalisation, adaptation, retention and maintenance.

Design prototypes

The way we sense the world is the way we understand the world. The caring practitioner needs to have a firm understanding of how the participant senses the world. The assessment templates provide the practitioner with a logical approach to identifying where the participant is on the detection–recognition–differentiation continuum for each of the senses. The design prototypes then provide the practitioner with clear guidelines as to how to actively design the environment to match participant need. The practitioner needs to be able to design an environment that makes this match with participant ability before a sensory conversation can begin.

Chapter 10

Beginning a sensory conversation

Introduction

Once the participant acquires the ability to detect a sense experience and is able to demonstrate evidence of this detection then the caring practitioner has something concrete with which to start the communication process. This initial communication would simply involve the practitioner being aware of the participant's detection of a stimulus and alternatively being aware of the participant's absence of detection. The way the practitioner becomes aware of the participant's ability to detect a sense experience is through what Noddings calls 'engrossment' (see Chapter 5).

Engrossment is a state of continuing complete absorption in the participant where the practitioner is as open as possible to identifying what the participant is trying to communicate. As open as possible means in practice that the practitioner needs to be working with just one participant at a time. Such limiting of context is a particularly powerful way of helping to ensure that the message received is as accurate as possible. At this early stage the bulk of the sensory conversation lies with the caring practitioner. The participant is only aware of detecting the sense stimulation. Still, if we define communication as the sharing or exchanging of information between two people then this would place such sharing within the definition of rudimentary communication.

Pleasure, power and meaning

The process of the practitioner sharing the participant's enjoyment of the detection of the sense experience introduces the possibility of associative learning, a basic building block of communication. The association between the affective (in this case the participant's enjoyment) and the sense experience provides the basis for learning. To begin with this association is at the pre-acquisition stage, such as the use of Mere Exposure Theory in the story of José and the Tibetan singing bowl. Over time and with sufficient repetition, the participant begins to associate the pleasurable experience of detecting sense stimuli with the pleasure of being with the caring practitioner. This ability to associate one experience with another provides the key to the practitioner building rapport with the participant.

It is interesting to consider how the will to pleasure, will to power and will to meaning (see Chapter 7) link in with neuroplasticity (see Chapter 6). The participant's will to pleasure makes him or her more open to repeating the experience (see Chapter 3), which coincides with Hebb's law, the main principle of neuroplasticity: 'neurons that fire together wire together' (Doidge 2007, p. 63). The participant's will to power is activated as neurons that are used survive, strengthen and ready the participant for transition from detection to recognition. Recognition is a precursor of differentiation and meaning, which are in turn predicated on further neuroplastic strengthening of sensory pathways, building up the brain bridge.

For this transition to recognition to actually occur though there needs to be some form of social interaction, recognition being essentially a social construct. We learned in Chapter 1 that the need for social interaction is fundamental. It is this social interaction that helps to ignite the will to meaning and provide the tipping point that finally takes the participant from detection to recognition. This need for social interaction helps to explain why it is so important for the practitioner to establish a caring relationship with the participant from the start. It is this caring relationship that provides the mechanical advantage to enable the participant to make the sensory processing developmental transitions described in this book.

Each new sensory processing transition expands the participant's sensory vocabulary, the pool of experiences the practitioner can employ to reach the participant. As the participant moves from being able to detect a sense experience to being able to recognise it, there is a corresponding expansion in the participant's capacity for pleasure, power and meaning. This capacity provides the participant and the practitioner with a growing repertoire of communication potentialities. The important point for the practitioner to remember though is that the participant can only consciously share what he or she is already able to experience. Any experience outside the participant's actual experiential repertoire may not be detected. The practitioner therefore is advised to keep precise records detailing the participant's achievements and to deliberately use this sensory vocabulary when communicating with the participant.

In Chapter 5 I talked about McLuhan's observation that the message is embedded in the medium, that the medium and the message have a symbiotic relationship. The caring practitioner therefore needs to be alert that the sharing that occurs with the participant is not only concerned with the overt message, but it is also aimed at helping the participant become aware of what it means to be cared for, to be part of a caring relationship. The goal is to reach a point in the participant's development where the participant is able to demonstrate recognition that an act of caring is taking place. Noddings argues that this cared-for state provides the optimum environment for learning and development to occur. It is when the conversation is ready to begin in earnest.

A conversation is defined as a succession of exchanges between two people where there is a sharing of information plus the possibility of new knowledge being generated. For communication to occur a channel must be opened between the two participants and some level of common ground established. In the case of the participant this common ground comprises the participant's sensory vocabulary. When the participant engages in an interaction and the practitioner observes it, the next step is for the practitioner to change the inter-action in some way that will be recognised and appreciated by the participant. For this to happen though both the participant and the practitioner must be fully attentive to what is happening between them. The moment this focused attention is removed, the conversation falters.

Practitioners support communication by being particularly alert to three aspects of the participant's communication. The first is to allow sufficient time for the participant to recognise and demonstrate appreciation. Practitioners need to take care not to allow themselves to be distracted by other priorities and issues that are not relevant to the participant. Allowing sufficient time for interaction is especially important when starting a conversation with the participant for the very first time. In participants with substantial brain damage the amount of time required for the participant to recognise and demonstrate appreciation may be much, much longer than initially anticipated.

The second consideration is for the practitioner to be aware that the strength of the demonstration might be much, much fainter than initially anticipated. The practitioner therefore needs to temper his or her expectations and use engrossment to more accurately measure the participant's attentional capacity, information processing speed and behaviour capability.

A third significant consideration is for the practitioner to be aware of the tremendous 'bio-cost' to the participant, that is the amount of physical energy required to achieve a behaviour breakthrough, and to think about whether the reward justifies the effort. Once again the reward must come from the parti-cipant's own sensory repertoire and capacity to construct meaning from the encounter. It is most meaningful to the participant when the participant takes the lead in the conversation. As a consequence it takes time before a conversation can progress beyond the initial participant interaction, practitioner response and participant recognition. However even such a brief encounter holds the seeds of effective communication because the encounter creates a new relationship between the two, something that did not previously exist. A change has taken place. The way the participant and the practitioner interact with each other has begun to evolve.

When the participant does choose to continue the conversation, most probably the participant will repeat the same initial interaction. The practitioner may then either copy it or repeat his or her previous interaction. In this way the conversation reaches an important new level of confirmation of understanding. The practitioner needs to work within the guidelines set down by the participant and initially be careful not to go outside these two options otherwise the participant will be confused, possibly overwhelmed.

Only when this sensory conversation is well established can the caring practitioner introduce appropriate new elements further along the detection–recognition–differentiation continuum.

Chapter 11

Extending the conversation

Introduction

Once the participant is able to successfully engage in an extended sensory conversation he or she is ready for the generation of new knowledge. Four ways to generate this new knowledge within the conversation are: modelling, dialogue, practice and confirmation (see Figure 11.1).

Even though these four actions have already been described (see Chapter 5), they will now be revisited as part of Social Learning Theory. This is the major turning point of the unified approach to using multisensory stimulation because this is where the participant changes from being passive to becoming active.

Social Learning Theory is based on the premise that learning takes place within a social context. It is therefore particularly germane to the unified approach. Social interactions underpin the sensory conversation between the caring professional and the participant. Social interactions are critical for neuroplasticity (see Chapter 6) and for sense development transitions along the

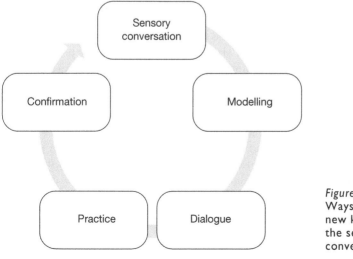

Figure 11.1
Ways to generate new knowledge in the sensory conversation.

detection–recognition–differentiation continuum (see Chapter 10). Social context plays the singular most important role in enabling us to make sense of the world (see Chapter 1) and shaping who we are.

The assumption behind Social Learning Theory is that learning involves both external stimuli and internal mechanisms. The theory is a bridge between Behaviorism, which assumes learning is the result of stimuli in the external environment, and Cognitivism, which assumes learning is a result of internal changes in a person's conceptual framework or schemata. Both types of learning occur to a greater or lesser extent depending on the circumstances.

Modelling

Bandura (1962, 1971), an advocate of Social Learning Theory, coined the term 'modeling' to explain how an individual observes a novel behaviour performed by another person, retains that behaviour and then replicates it to make it their own. Synonyms variously used for modelling are 'vicarious learning', 'social learning' and 'imitation'.

For Bandura (1977) modelling has four preconditions, namely: attention, retention, reproduction and motivation. While the caring professional tries to nurture all four conditions, motivation is especially significant. This is because it is motivation that transforms the participant from being passive into becoming an active participant in the sensory conversation (Sirkkola and Pagliano 2009).

Earlier (see Chapter 7) I drew attention to the Sapir–Whorf hypothesis, the idea that the structure of the language we use strongly moulds our conception of the world. Moreover I drew parallels and argued that the way we use our senses to engage with the world strongly moulds our conception of the world. This point is particularly relevant for modelling. The caring practitioner must use the sensory vocabulary of the participant, not the caring practitioner's own, in order for the participant to be able to derive the most meaning from the modelling.

This is particularly relevant in regard to vision and to a lesser extent hearing. Hart (1987, p. 391) estimates that 'about 80% of learning takes place through the visual modality', which may suit those with vision, but it provides substantial learning and developmental challenges for participants who do not learn through the visual modality. As Swallow (1988, p. 5) points out: 'Visual loss profoundly affects the socialisation process' and it greatly reduces natural opportunities for vicarious learning. The same can be said about hearing. The test for the caring practitioner then is to work out how, using the sense abilities that are available to that participant, to provide models that can be recognised and imitated. For this to happen, the caring practitioner must somehow switch off his or her own way of experiencing the world and become fully engrossed in determining how the participant experiences the world.

Karen's interaction with Suzette helps to illustrate how such a modelling process might take place. In addition to profound intellectual disability and physical impairment, three-year-old Suzette has very little functional vision and very little functional hearing. She therefore has profound multiple disabilities. Karen, her caring practitioner, decided to model a sensory conversation using a sensory vocabulary from the senses of interoception, chemosensation and the somatic senses. However even these senses are limited because of Suzette's physical impairment. The situation is compounded by Suzette being fed via a percutaneous endoscopic gastrostomy (PEG) tube (i.e. limited taste experiences) and by her extreme lack of sensory stimulation generally up to this point in time.

Karen always starts her sensory conversation with a gentle touch just below Suzette's bottom lip, which mostly results in a slight smile of recognition. It took quite a while for Karen to even perfect this initial greeting. Karen then puts her hand on Suzette's hand and gives it a little squeeze and waits once again for Suzette to respond with another slight smile of recognition. Once again this took many sessions to achieve. Next Karen puts her hand in Suzette's hand and waits for Suzette to respond with a diminutive squeeze of her own. It took five sessions before Suzette, ever so slightly, squeezed back. When this first happened, Karen in her excitement gave Suzette another gentle touch just below her bottom lip as a reward. Karen's exhilaration came from the fact that Suzette had freely chosen to copy her behaviour. Karen reported: 'Suzette being willing and able to imitate me was such a great honour. After all the work I've done with her I now feel like the tide is beginning to turn.'

Dialogue

The second way to enrich a conversation is through dialogue. At first it might seem incongruous to make a distinction between conversation and dialogue; however for the purposes of this book conversation is merely a succession of exchanges where information is shared whereas dialogue is more refined, more sophisticated. Noddings describes dialogue as a style of interaction, which grows out of engrossment where the carer models caring by trying to understand the cared-for's communication motive and just as importantly the participant's communication sense vocabulary.

The Russian semiotician Bakhtin (1986) goes further. For him dialogue has the power to provide the communicator with a different perspective, one that forces change. With true dialogue there is equality between the participants and both are active. This is a tremendously important point when the dialogue is between a caring practitioner and a participant, especially considering how so many people with profound multiple disabilities spend so much of their lives being done to and passive, unequal. Dialogue therefore is different to conversation, because dialogue is a political concept where the power to force change is defined by 'the human ability . . . to act in concert' (Arendt 1972, p. 143). The caring practitioner and the participant work as one.

It is interesting to consider this interpretation of dialogue in the context of Williams' (1998) description of not being aware of the difference between herself and the sensory experience and also in the context of Mahler *et al.*'s (1975) description of 'a normal autistic phase' (see Chapter 4). Dialogue helps to explain how the caring practitioner might use communication as a vehicle to generate change in participant awareness.

Returning to Suzette, Karen discovered that if, in addition to her own modelling, she copied Suzette, then this provided her with greater insight into what behaviours Suzette could engage in. It helped her to build up her understanding of Suzette's sensory vocabulary. Karen also discovered that modelling those behaviours back to Suzette provided Suzette with a new opportunity for her to observe her own behaviour. So Karen gave a gentle squeeze to Suzette's hand a second time and then put her hand inside Suzette's hand to wait for her to repeat the behaviour.

If we return to Halliday's triptych (see Chapter 4) we can see that the above dialogue between Karen and Suzette ensures that Suzette is not only learning 'of' her sense vocabulary and subsequently 'through' her sense vocabulary but also learning 'about' the sense vocabulary. This early meta-sense ability might be what is needed to eventually help Suzette move out of the normal autistic stage and start to see herself as separate to her sense experience. Of course Karen realises that she still has a lot of work to do with Suzette before such a change eventuates. It will entail time, patience and plenty of practice.

Practice

For Noddings (1984) practice is where the cared-for gains mastery over his or her behavioural repertoire. She describes it as being involved in a caring apprenticeship so the practice takes place within the sensory conversation, when it has achieved a level of dialogue and in conjunction with modelling. This idea of apprenticeship is similar to Vygotsky's Social Development Theory, which is based on the assumption that social interaction comes before learning (Vygotsky 1978). Vygotsky's theory offers a radical departure from Piaget's understanding that development precedes learning (Piaget 1928). Social Development Theory is built on two accompanying principles, both known by their acronyms: MKO and ZPD. MKO stands for the 'more knowledgeable other' who in this case is the caring practitioner and ZPD stands for 'zone of proximal development'. ZPD is defined as the distance between what the participant is able to independently achieve and what the participant is able to achieve with support from the MKO. The MKO is able to change the level of support by adjusting the available scaffolding. Karen did this with Suzette. At first she would put her hand in Suzette's hand and then put her other hand over Suzette's hand and squeeze Suzette's hand so Suzette's hand would then squeeze hers, then she would repeat the behaviour without the scaffold.

Confirmation

The fourth way to generate new knowledge is through what Noddings calls confirmation. This is where the caring practitioner provides the participant with a special type of corroborative feedback. The practitioner offers the participant a new kind of evidence or additional proof that the behaviour was recognised and appreciated. It is therefore the final part of the practitioner apprenticeship relationship. Noddings (1984, p. 193) says: 'When we attribute the best possible motive consonant with reality to the cared-for, we confirm.' However for the caring practitioner to be able to provide consistent, high quality, precise and meaningful confirmation to the participant there must be ongoing engrossment. The moment the practitioner ceases to give his or her very best attention and empathy to the participant then the validation loses its potency.

Chapter 12

Catching the wave

Introduction

Discipline-centred techniques are generally developed in the much larger population of people with disabilities who have no need of targeted multisensory stimulation. The overwhelming body of literature validating the use of these techniques therefore relates to this majority population. Discipline-specific literature in the participant group with severe sensory disabilities is sparse. This is because these participants are on the far lower edge of the disability population bell curve. They are as different from one another as they are from the majority population.

The usual approach adopted by each discipline has been to extrapolate back the techniques so successfully used for other participants with less severe disabilities. For the participants with a severe sensory disability however, this approach has been at best hit and miss, often hindered by the difficulty of measuring outcomes using conventional discipline measures.

The unified approach puts a primary focus on actively working at the sensory thresholds of the participant, using the ideas, tools and approaches elaborated in this book. The success or not of an intervention is primarily defined in sensory threshold terms. This is because without sensory perceptual development there can be no other meaningful development. Success of an intervention defined in conventional discipline terms is hard to interpret without this multisensory focus.

However the context in which unified approach interventions occur is discipline-specific, dependent on the background and expertise of the practitioner. As a result, ongoing professional development encompasses two strands, those relating to multisensory issues and those relating to discipline-specific issues. The two are complementary but hierarchical, multisensory having primacy over discipline-specific. This necessitates a major reconceptualisation of priorities within each discipline when addressing issues relating to this particular participant group.

Considered reflection is the cornerstone of exemplary professional practice, whatever the field. In the context of the practitioner working with participants using multisensory stimulation, it is pivotal. Returning to the discipline for extension work is essential to keep techniques up-to-date, refined and skilful.

New techniques are constantly being developed and these can further enrich practice. Developing high precision is the crux so multisensory participant interventions take the form intended.

Once the caring practitioner is able to successfully conduct a sensory conversation with the participant and extend that conversation through modelling, dialogue, practice and confirmation then the participant is more ready to be served by practitioners from a range of other different specialist disciplines. Liaising *within* discipline boundaries with other caring practitioners can help improve the seamless intertwining of the multisensory and discipline-specific strands. Liaising *across* discipline boundaries to confer on multisensory approaches can profoundly help revitalise professional practice.

The unified approach benefits from discipline-specific insights. Disciplines benefit from insights from practitioners working with participants using multisensory stimulation using the unified approach. The participants do not then become the forlorn, silent forgotten minority they would be otherwise, dumped in the 'too hard' basket.

Catching the wave

I want to end this book on a high note, to show just how exciting using the unified approach can be. Initially when addressing detection and recognition thresholds, the sensory conversation tends to be tenuous and tentative as vocabulary is laid down. The conversation morphs more easily into the deeper richer sensory dialogue when differentiation thresholds are being addressed. It is akin to the surfing metaphor, catching the wave.

One approach I like was developed by Linda Messbauer (2011). It involves three steps. The first step is called 'Wow'. This is where the caring practitioner designs sensory stimulation just right for the participant's stage of sense development. The participant is sufficiently captivated by the stimulation to become fascinated (see Chapter 4). Fascination indicates that the participant is finding the sense experience gratifying and it is this gratification that strongly motivates the participant to want to continue to engage with the stimulation. Typical fascination follows an engagement curve where the attention goes up, plateaus for a while and then subsides.

The second step is called 'Modulation'. When the fascination is subsiding, the intensity of the stimulation is changed by the caring practitioner to re-arouse fascination again. During these two stages the participant remains passive. The stimulation is made freely available to the participant and the participant experiences an abundance of sensory success (see Chapter 3). Once again, the re-aroused fascination is allowed to follow an engagement curve – the attention goes up, plateaus for a while and then subsides.

The third step is called 'Exercise'. When the modulated fascination subsides, the caring practitioner changes the stimulation again – this time to entice the participant to become active in some way in order to seek out fascination from the stimulus again. For example if the participant is visually motivated, an interesting light source might be moved so as to require the participant to turn his or her head to see it. Once the participant is actively engaging with the stimulation then the participant is making what is termed an adapted response (see Chapter 9).

Adaptive responses provide the basis of more sophisticated sensory conversations and dialogue. They promote an internal locus of control. They can be used to redirect stereotypies. They are the entry point into conventional mainstream disability interventions and techniques. Once the stage of adaptive responses has been reached, the wave can move quickly, vastly expanding the sensory world of the participant.

This is the goal of the unified approach and the culmination of all the groundwork laid down throughout this book. I hope I have inspired you.

References

Abitz, M., Nielsen, R. D., Jones, E. G., Laursen, H., Graem, N. and Pakkenberg, B. (2007) Excess of neurons in the human newborn mediodorsal thalamus compared with that of the adult. *Cerebral Cortex*, 17 (11), pp. 2573–2578.

Adler, A. (1956) *The individual psychology of Alfred Adler: a systematic presentation in selections from his writings* (eds Ansbacher, H. L. and Ansbacher, R. R.). New York: Harper Torchbooks.

Ananthakrishnan, T. and Sen, A. (eds) (1998) *Biocommunication in insects*. Enfield, CT: Science Publishers Inc.

Arendt, H. (1972) *On violence in crises in the republic*. Orlando, FL: Harcourt Brace and Company.

Bandura, A. (1962) Social learning through imitation. In: Jones, M. R. (ed.) *Nebraska symposium on motivation*. Lincoln, NE: University of Nebraska Press, pp. 211–269.

Bandura, A. (1971) *Psychological modeling: conflicting theories*. New York: Aldine-Atherton.

Bandura, A. (1977) *Social Learning Theory*. Englewood Cliffs, NJ: Prentice Hall.

Bakhtin, M. M. (1986) *Speech genres and other late essays*. Trans. by McGee, V. W. Austin, TX: University of Texas Press.

Bennett, R. (2011) *Virtual worlds offer opportunities for people with disabilities*. [Online] Available from: http://www.disaboom.com/assistive-technology-general/virtual-worlds-offer-opportunities-for-people-with-disabilities [Accessed 30/09/11].

Blesser, B. and Salter, L.-R. (2007) *Spaces speak, are you listening? Experiencing aural architecture*. Cambridge, MA: MIT Press.

Bly, L. (1983) *Components of normal development during the first year of life and abnormal development*. [Monograph] Oak Park, IL: Neurodevelopmental Treatment Association.

Brown, D. (2002/2003) Resonance boards, deaf-blind perspectives. *Deaf-Blind Perspectives*, 10 (2) [Online] Available at: http://www.nationaldb.org/dbp/dec2002.htm [Accessed 30/09/11].

Bunning, K. (1996) Development of an 'Individualised Sensory Environment' for adults with learning difficulties and an evaluation of its effects on their interactive behaviours. Unpublished thesis, London City University.

Bunning, K. (1998) To engage or not to engage: affecting the interactions of learning disabled adults. *International Journal of Language and Communication Disorders*, 33, pp. 368–391.

Calvert, G., Spence, C. and Stein, B. (eds) (2004) *The handbook of multisensory processes*. Cambridge, MA: MIT Press.

Clark, A. (2008) *Supersizing the mind: embodiment, action, and cognitive extension*. Oxford: Oxford University Press.

Clark, A. (2011) Predictive Coding. What scientific concept would improve everybody's cognitive toolkit? [Online] Available from: http://www.edge.org/q2011/q11_6.html [Accessed 30/09/11].

Classen, C. (2005) McLuhan in the rainforest: the sensory worlds of oral cultures. In: Howes, D. (ed.) *Empire of the senses: the sensual culture reader*. Oxford: Berg, pp. 147–163.

Cleland, C. C. and Clark, C. M. (1966) Sensory deprivation and aberrant behavior among idiots. *American Journal of Mental Deficiency*, 71, pp. 213–393.

Csikszentmihalyi, M. (1990) *Flow: the psychology of optimal experience*. New York: Harper and Row.

Csikszentmihalyi, M. (1998) *Finding flow: the psychology of engagement with everyday life*. New York: Basic Books.

Danesi, M. (1994) *Messages and meanings: an introduction to Semiotics*. Toronto, ON: Canadian Scholars' Press.

DeGrandpre, R. (2000) *Ritalin nation: rapid fire culture and the transformation of human consciousness*. New York: Norton Paperback.

Dell'Orto, S. (2003) W.D. Winnicott and the transitional object in infancy. *Pediatric Medicine Chirurgic*, 25 (2), pp. 106–112.

Deshpande, D. A., Wang, W. C. H., McIlmoyle, E. L., Robinett, K. S., Schillinger, R. M., An, S. S. *et al.* (2010) Bitter taste receptors on airway smooth muscle bronchodilate by localized calcium signaling and reverse obstruction. *Nature Medicine*, 16, pp. 1299–1304.

Doidge, N. (2007) *The brain that changes itself: stories of personal triumph from the frontiers of brain science*. New York: Viking (Penguin).

Dubuc, B. (2002) The brain from top to bottom: the evolutionary layers of the human brain. [Online] Available from: http://thebrain.mcgill.ca/flash/d/d_05/d_05_cr/d_05_cr_her/d_05_cr_her.html [Accessed 30/09/11].

Erikson, E. H. (1950) *Childhood and society*. New York: Norton.

Frankl, V. [1946] (2006) *Man's search for meaning*. Boston: Beacon Press.

Flannery, R. B. Jr (2002) Treating learned helplessness in the elderly dementia patient: preliminary inquiry. *American Journal of Alzheimer's Disease and Other Dementias*, 17 (6), pp. 345–349.

Fleming, N. (2010) How kids get grown-up vision. *New Scientist*, 208 (2784), p. 19.

Freud, S. (1920) *Beyond the pleasure principle* (Jenseits des Lustprinzips). [Online] Available from: http://www.gutenberg.org/browse/authors/f - a391 [Accessed 30/09/11].

Frisch, K. von. (1967) *The dance language and orientation of bees*. Cambridge, MA: The Belknap Press of Harvard University Press.

Fuad-Luke, A. (2004) *Slow theory – a paradigm for living sustainably?* [Online] Available from: www.slowdesign.org/pdf/Slow%20design.pdf [Accessed 30/09/11].

Garner, J. P. (2005) Stereotypies and other abnormal repetitive behaviors: potential impact on validity, reliability, and replicability of scientific outcomes. *ILAR (Institute for Laboratory Animal Research) Journal*, 46 (2), pp. 106–117.

Gibson, J. J. (1966) *The senses considered as perceptual systems*. Boston: Houghton Mifflin.

Gibson, J. J. (1977) The theory of affordances. In: Shaw, R. and Bransford, J. (eds) *Perceiving, acting, and knowing: toward an ecological psychology*. Hillsdale, NJ: Lawrence Erlbaum, pp. 67–82.

Gladwell, M. (2000) *The tipping point: how little things can make a big difference*. London: Abacus.

Greason, P. B. and Cashwell, C. S. (2009) Mindfulness and counseling self-efficacy: the mediating role of attention and empathy. *Counselor Education and Supervision*, 49 (1), pp. 2–19.

Gregory, R. L. (1970) *The intelligent eye*. London: Weidenfeld and Nicolson.

Gusky, T. R. and Gates, S. (1986) Synthesis of research on the effects of mastery learning in elementary and secondary classrooms. *Educational Leadership*, 43, pp. 73–80.

Halliday, M. A. K. (1979) Language development project. Occasional paper. Canberra, ACT: Curriculum Development Centre.

Halliday, M. A. K. (1993) Towards a learning-based theory of language. *Linguistics and Education*, 5, pp. 93–116.

Hart, V. (1987) Developmental differences in vision. In: Neisworth, J. T. and Bagnato, S. T. (eds) *The young exceptional child: early education and development*. New York: Macmillan, pp. 388–413.

Hines, R. M., Wu, L., Hines, D. J., Steenland, H., Mansour, S., Dahlhaus, R. et al. (2008) Synaptic imbalance, stereotypies, and impaired social interactions in mice with altered neuroligin expression. *The Journal of Neuroscience*, 28 (24) pp. 6055–6067.

Hoijer, H. (ed.) (1954) *Language in culture: conference on the interrelations of language and other aspects of culture*. Chicago, MA: University of Chicago Press.

Hull, J. M. (2000) Blindness and the face of God: toward a theology of disability. In: Ziebertz, H., Schweitzer, F., Häring, H. and Browning, D. (eds) *The human image of God*. Leiden, The Netherlands: Brill, pp. 215–229.

Hulsegge, J. and Verheul, A. (1986; Dutch 1987; English translation by R. Alink) *Snoezelen another world: a practical book of sensory experience environments for the mentally handicapped*. Chesterfield: ROMPA.

Jones, M. C. (1924) A laboratory study of fear: the case of Peter. *The Pedagogical Seminary*, 31, pp. 308–315.

Joseph, R. (1999) Environmental influences on neural plasticity, the limbic system, emotional development and attachment: a review. *Child Psychiatry and Human Development*, 29 (3), pp. 189–208.

Jütte, R. (2005) *A history of the senses: from antiquity to cyberspace*. Cambridge: Polity Press.

Kellert, S. H. (1993) *In the wake of chaos: unpredictable order in dynamical systems*. Chicago: University of Chicago Press.

Klein, S. (2002; English translation by S. Lehmann) *The science of happiness: how our brains make us happy – and what we can do to get happier*. New York: Marlowe and Co. (Avalon Publishing Group).

Koluchova, J. (1972) Severe deprivation in twins: a case study. *Journal of Child Psychology and Psychiatry*, 13, pp. 107–114.

Koluchova, J. (1976) The further development of twins after severe and prolonged deprivation: a second report. *Journal of Child Psychology and Psychiatry*, 17, pp. 181–188.

Korsmeyer, C. (1998) *Aesthetics: the big question*. Oxford: Blackwell Publishing.

Kozloff, M. A. and Rice, J. S. (1998) *Parent and family issues: stress and knowledge*. [Online] Available from: http://www/uncwll.edu/people/kozloffm/family autism.html [Accessed 11/03/2001].

Kuhl, P. (2007) Is speech learning 'gated' by the social brain? *Developmental Science*, 10 (1), pp. 110–120.

Kuhn, T. S. (1996) *The structure of scientific revolutions*. 3rd ed. Chicago: University of Chicago Press.

Lin Lu, Guobin Bao, Hai Chen, Peng Xia, Xueliang Fan, Jisheng Zhang, *et al.* (2003) Modification of hippocampal neurogenesis and neuroplasticity by social environments. *Experimental Neurology*, 183 (2), pp. 600–609.

Linden, D. (2007) *The accidental mind: how brain evolution has given us love, memory, dreams, and God*. Cambridge, MA: Belknap Press of the Harvard University Press.

Lorenz, K. (1952) *King Solomon's ring*. New York: Crowell.

MacLean, P. D. (1990) *The Triune brain in evolution: Role of Paleocerebral functions*. New York: Springer.

McLuhan, M. (1961) Inside the five sense sensorium. *The Canadian Architect*, 6, pp. 49–54.

McLuhan, M. (1964) *Understanding media: the extensions of man*. New York: McGraw Hill.

Mahler, M. S., Pine, R. and Bergmann, A. (1975) *The psychological birth of the human infant: symbiosis and individuation*. New York: Basic Books.

Marstaller, L. (2009) Review – supersizing the mind. Embodiment, action, and cognitive extension by Andy Clark. *Metapsychology Online Reviews*, 13 (10) [Online] Available from: http://metapsychology.mentalhelp.net/poc/view_doc.php?type=book&id=4795&cn=396 [Accessed 30/09/11].

Maslow, A. (1954) *Motivation and personality*. New York: Harper.

Mertens, K. (2008) *Snoezelen – in action*. Aachen, Germany: Shaker Verlag.

Messbauer, L. (2011) *Multi-sensory environments*. [Online] Available at: http://lmessbauer.com/ [Accessed 30/09/11].

Neisworth, J. T. and Bagnato, S. J. (1988) Assessment in early childhood special education: a typology of dependent measures. In: Odom, S. L. and Karnes, M. B. (eds) *Early intervention for infants and children with handicaps: an empirical base*. Baltimore MD: Paul H. Brookes Publishing, pp. 23–51.

Nielsen, L. (1992) *Educational approaches for visually impaired children*. Copenhagen: Sikon.

Noddings, N. (1984) *Caring: a feminine approach to ethics and moral education*. Berkeley, CA: University of California Press.

Noddings, N. (1992) *The challenge to care in schools: an alternative approach to education* (Advances in contemporary educational thought series, vol. 8). New York: Teachers College Press.

Noddings, N. (1995) *Philosophy of education* (Dimensions of philosophy series). Boulder, CO: Westview Press.

Ong, W. J. (1969) World as view and world as event. *American Anthropologist*, 71 (4), pp. 634–647.

Oxford dictionaries (2011) Oxford: Oxford University Press [Online] Available from: http://oxforddictionaries.com/definition/communication [Accessed 30.09.11].

Pagliano, P. J. (1999) *Multisensory environments*. London: David Fulton Publishers.

Pagliano, P. J. (2001) *Using a multisensory environment: a practical guide for teachers*. London: David Fulton.

Peirce, C. S. (1931–1958) *Collected writings* (8 Vols.) (eds Hartshorne, C., Weiss, P. and Burks, A. W.). Cambridge, MA: Harvard University Press.

Perry, B. D. and Pollard, R. (1997) Altered brain development following global neglect in early childhood. In: *Proceedings from the Society for Neuroscience Annual Meeting.* New Orleans: The Society for Neuroscience.

Piaget, J. (1928) *The child's conception of the world.* London: Routledge and Kegan Paul.

Poppes, P., van der Putten, A. J. J. and Vlaskamp, C. (2010) Frequency and severity of challenging behaviour in people with profound intellectual and multiple disabilities. *Research in Developmental Disabilities,* 31, pp. 1269–1275.

Posit Science Companion Guide (2005–2007) Posit Science, San Francisco, CA.

Ratey. J. (2001) *A user's guide to the brain.* London: Abacus.

Rogers, C. (1957) The necessary and sufficient conditions of therapeutic personality change. *Journal of Consulting Psychology,* 21 (2), pp. 95–103

Rogers, R. (1997) *Cities for a small planet.* London: Faber & Faber Ltd.

Sacks, O. (2005) *The mind's eye: what the blind see.* In: Howes, D. (ed.) *Empire of the senses: the sensual culture reader.* Oxford: Berg, pp. 25–42.

Sebeok, T. (ed.) (1977) *How animals communicate.* Bloomington, IN: Indiana University Press.

Seligman, M. E. P. (1975) *Helplessness: on depression, development, and death.* San Francisco, CA: W. H. Freeman.

Seligman, M. E. P. (1998) *Learned optimism.* New York: Pocket Books.

Seligman, M. E. P. and Maier, S. F. (1967) Failure to escape traumatic shock. *Journal of Experimental Psychology,* 74, pp. 1–9.

Shannon, C. E. and Weaver, W. (1949) *A mathematical model of communication.* Urbana, IL: University of Illinois Press

Sirkkola, M. and Pagliano, P. J. (2009) Increasing the level of participation in individuals with vision impairment and multiple disabilities: an analysis of the Multisensory Environment literature. *Journal of the South Pacific Educators in Vision Impairment,* 4 (1), pp. 15–24.

Spitz, R. A. (1945) Hospitalism: an inquiry into the genesis of psychiatric conditions in early childhood. *Psychoanalytical Study Child,* 1, pp. 53–74.

Stone, J. V. (2011) Footprints sticking out of the sand. Part 2: Children's Bayesian priors for shape and lighting direction. *Perception,* 40 (2), pp. 175–190.

Stone, J. V. and Pascalis, O. (2010) Footprints sticking out of the sand. Part 1: Children's perception of naturalistic and embossed symbol stimuli. *Perception,* 39 (9), pp. 1254–1260.

South, E. M. (2001) *The effects of graduated exposure, modeling and contingent attention on tolerance to skin care products with children with autism.* Master of Science thesis, University of North Texas. [Online] Available from: http://digital.library.unt.edu/ark:/67531/metadc3028/ [Accessed 30/09/11].

Swallow, R. (1988) Lifelong learning: future directions in the education of children with visual disabilities. In: *Tomorrow today. Proceedings of the ANZAEVH Biennial Conference.* Melbourne, Victoria: The Association.

Turner, W. D., Realon, R. E., Irvin, D. and Robinson, E. (1996) The effects of implementing program consequences with a group of individuals who engaged in sensory maintained hand mouthing. *Research in Developmental Disabilities,* 17 (4), pp. 311–330.

United Nations (2011) [1948] The universal declaration of human rights. [Online] Available from: http://www.un.org/en/documents/udhr/ [Accessed 30/09/11].

Verheul, A. (2007) *Snoezelen materials homemade*. Ede, The Netherlands: Ad Verheul.

Vos, P., De Cock, P., Petry, K., Van Den Noortgate, W. and Maes, B. (2010) What makes them feel like they do? Investigating the subjective well-being in people with severe and profound disabilities. *Research in Developmental Disabilities*, 31, pp. 1623–1632.

Vygotsky, L. S. (1978) *Mind and society: the development of higher mental processes*. Cambridge, MA: Harvard University Press.

Weinstock, G. M. *et al.* (2006) Insights into social insects from the genome of the honeybee Apis mellifera. *Nature*, 443, pp. 931–949.

Williams, D. (1998) *Autism and sensing: the unlost instinct*. London: Jessica Kingsley.

Williams, D. L., Goldstein G. and Minshew, N. J. (2006) Profile of memory function in children with autism. *Neuropsychology*, 20, pp. 21–29.

Winnicott, D. W. (1971) *Playing and reality*. London: Routledge.

Wolpe, J. (1958) *Psychotherapy by reciprocal inhibition*. Stanford, CA: Stanford University Press.

Wright, B. A. (1960) *Physical disability: a psychological approach*. New York: Harper & Row.

Zajonc, R. B. (1968) Attitudinal effects of mere exposures. *Journal of Personality and Social Psychology*, 9 (2 Pt. 2), pp. 1–27.

Zajonc, R. B. (2001) Mere exposure: a gateway to the subliminal. *Current Directions in Psychological Science*, 10 (6), pp. 224–228.

Index